FREE Study Skills DVD Offer

Dear Customer,

Thank you for your purchase from Mometrix! We consider it an honor and a privilege that you have purchased our product and we want to ensure your satisfaction.

As a way of showing our appreciation and to help us better serve you, we have developed a Study Skills DVD that we would like to give you for <u>FREE</u>. This DVD covers our *best practices* for getting ready for your exam, from how to use our study materials to how to best prepare for the day of the test.

All that we ask is that you email us with feedback that would describe your experience so far with our product. Good, bad, or indifferent, we want to know what you think!

To get your FREE Study Skills DVD, email <u>freedvd@mometrix.com</u> with *FREE STUDY SKILLS DVD* in the subject line and the following information in the body of the email:

- The name of the product you purchased.
- Your product rating on a scale of 1-5, with 5 being the highest rating.
- Your feedback. It can be long, short, or anything in between. We just want to know your impressions and experience so far with our product. (Good feedback might include how our study material met your needs and ways we might be able to make it even better. You could highlight features that you found helpful or features that you think we should add.)
- Your full name and shipping address where you would like us to send your free DVD.

If you have any questions or concerns, please don't hesitate to contact me directly.

Thanks again!

Sincerely,

Jay Willis
Vice President
jay.willis@mometrix.com
1-800-673-8175

D1191244

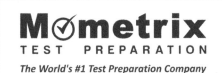

Mometrix
TEST PREPARATION
The World's #1 Test Preparation Company

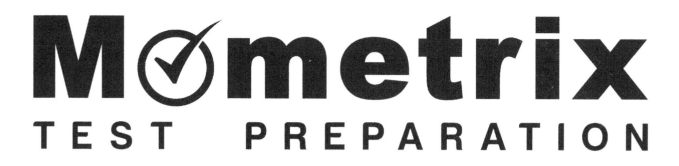

NCLEX PN
2019
Practice Questions

**3 NCLEX PN Examination Practice Tests
For the National Council Licensure
Examination for Practical
Nurses**

Written and edited by the Mometrix Nursing Certification Test Team

Printed in the United States of America

This paper meets the requirements of ANSI/NISO Z39.48-1992 (Permanence of Paper).

Mometrix offers volume discount pricing to institutions. For more information or a price quote, please contact our sales department at sales@mometrix.com or 888-248-1219.

Mometrix Media LLC is not affiliated with or endorsed by any official testing organization. All organizational and test names are trademarks of their respective owners.

ISBN 13: 978-1-5167-1141-3
ISBN 10: 1-5167-1141-6

DEAR FUTURE EXAM SUCCESS STORY

First of all, **THANK YOU** for purchasing Mometrix study materials!

Second, congratulations! You are one of the few determined test-takers who are committed to doing whatever it takes to excel on your exam. **You have come to the right place.** We developed these practice tests with one goal in mind: to deliver you the best possible approximation of the questions you will see on test day.

Standardized testing is one of the biggest obstacles on your road to success, which only increases the importance of doing well in the high-pressure, high-stakes environment of test day. Your results on this test could have a significant impact on your future, and these practice tests will give you the repetitions you need to build your familiarity and confidence with the test content and format to help you achieve your full potential on test day.

Your success is our success

We would love to hear from you! If you would like to share the story of your exam success or if you have any questions or comments in regard to our products, please contact us at **800-673-8175** or **support@mometrix.com**.

Thanks again for your business and we wish you continued success!

Sincerely,
The Mometrix Test Preparation Team

TABLES OF CONTENTS

Practice Test #1

1. A client who has denied drug allergies has a telephone order for IM penicillin. Before the nurse administers the medication, the client states he thinks he may have developed a rash after "some drug." Which is the correct action?

    1. administer the drug and document a possible previous drug reaction
    2. hold the drug and contact the prescribing physician
    3. contact the pharmacist for guidance
    4. contact the supervisor for guidance

2. Which of the following blood products is indicated for a client with disseminated intravascular coagulation (DIC) to control bleeding where replacement of coagulation factors is necessary?

    1. whole blood
    2. irradiated red blood cells
    3. fresh frozen plasma
    4. platelets (multiple donors)

3. A client has requested pain medication, but after the nurse obtains the prescribed dose of codeine from the dispensing cart, the client refuses to take the medication, stating he might want it later. What should the nurse do with the medication?

    1. return it to the dispensing cart
    2. leave it at the client's bedside
    3. dispose of the medication according to facility protocol with two appropriate witnesses
    4. place the medication in a tray for later use

4. With a drop factor of 15 drops per 1 mL, what drip rate should the nurse set to deliver 1000 mL of intravenous D5W in 3 hours and 20 minutes? *Record your answer using a whole number.*

5. A client with vaginal cancer is being treated with brachytherapy, and the nurse is explaining the procedure and precautions to the client. Which of the following information should the nurse include?

    1. "Women who are pregnant and children under age 18 may not visit."
    2. "Visitors should stay at least 2 feet away from the client."
    3. "You can only leave your room for 5 to 10 minutes per day."
    4. "Visitors can stay no more than 4 hours per day."

6. When preparing to do a sterile dressing change, the nurse places sterile gauze pads on the sterile field but inadvertently touches the sterile field with an ungloved hand. Which of the following should the nurse do next?

    1. use only gauze pads from the sterile field away from the contaminated area
    2. discard the gauze pads and sterile field and start over
    3. continue with dressing change, as the gauze pads were not contaminated
    4. place a new sterile field and using sterile gloves take gauze pads from the contaminated field and place on the new field

7. If a medication is available at 100 mg per 10 mL, how many milliliters does a dose of 120 mg require? *Record your* answer *using a whole number.*

8. A client comes to the doctor's office with a first-degree sprained ankle. Which of the following treatments does the nurse anticipate?

    1. cast
    2. splint
    3. RICE (rest, ice, compression, elevation)
    4. surgical repair

9. While observing the team leader irrigating a PICC line, a new nurse notes that the team leader has broken aseptic technique and contaminated the irrigating syringe. Which of the following actions is most appropriate?

    1. report the team leader to a supervisor
    2. ask the team leader after the irrigation if sterile technique was required
    3. say nothing because the new nurse is inexperienced
    4. tell the team leader immediately that the irrigating syringe was contaminated

10. A client has experienced a cardiac arrest at an office visit and the nurse is going to administer defibrillation with an automated external defibrillator (AED). Which of the following should the nurse remove prior to administering a shock?

    1. client's watch
    2. client's bra with metal wires
    3. client's dentures
    4. client's nose ring

11. A 60-kg adult is to receive a medication that is administered at 0.5 mg per kg per 24 hours. If the medication is given in 2 equal doses (every 12 hours), how many milligrams should be in each dose? *Record your answer using a whole number.*

12. A client receiving digoxin exhibits tachycardia and complains of headache and fatigue, nausea, diarrhea, and halo vision. Which of the following is probably the cause?

    1. digoxin dosage too low
    2. allergic response to digoxin
    3. digoxin toxicity
    4. disorder unrelated to digoxin

13. When teaching a client with a seizure disorder about long-term use of phenytoin, the nurse should stress the necessity for which of the following? Select all that apply.

    1. dental care
    2. hearing examinations
    3. vitamin D therapy and evaluation for osteoporosis
    4. drug compliance
    5. regular exercise

14. A client is taking the loop diuretic furosemide for edema associated with heart failure. Which electrolyte imbalance resulting from the medication is of most concern?

1. hypokalemia
2. hyperkalemia
3. hypercalcemia
4. hypocalcemia

15. The nurse is teaching a newly diagnosed client with diabetes mellitus type 1 about self-care. Which of the following information should the nurse include? Select all that apply.

1. glucose testing
2. skin care
3. dietary compliance
4. bowel care
5. insulin administration

16. The nurse must administer eye drops to a 6-month-old infant, but the child clinches the eyes tightly to avoid the drops. Which of the following actions is the most appropriate?

1. attempt to instill the drops at a later time
2. force the infant's eyes open using the thumb and index finger
3. gently restrain the head and apply the drops at the inner canthus
4. pull down the lower lid with the thumb and instill the drops into the conjunctival sac

17. Which is the preferred site for intramuscular injections for both adults and children?

1. deltoid
2. ventrogluteal
3. dorsogluteal
4. vastus lateralis

18. A client is receiving a liter of normal saline intravenously but must receive 150 mL of antibiotic solution by piggyback. Which of the following is the most correct procedure?

1. clamp the primary tubing and adjust the flow rate of the piggyback unit
2. hang the piggyback unit 6 inches lower than the primary unit and adjust flow rate of the piggyback unit only
3. hang the piggyback unit 6 inches higher than the primary unit and adjust flow rate of the piggyback unit only
4. hang the piggyback unit at the same level as the primary unit, clamp the primary tubing, and adjust flow rate of the piggyback unit

19. Prior to administering an IV push medication, which of the following should the nurse check? Select all that apply.

1. dosage and correct dilution
2. recommended administration time
3. availability of pharmacist
4. client allergies
5. client's identification

Mometrix

20. How long should a woman remain in the supine position after administration of a vaginal suppository?

    1. 1 to 2 minutes
    2. 3 to 5 minutes
    3. 5 to 10 minutes
    4. 15 minutes

21. Which vitamin or mineral may alter the effect of levodopa in clients treated for Parkinson disease?

    1. calcium
    2. vitamin D
    3. ascorbic acid (Vitamin C)
    4. pyridoxine (Vitamin B6)

22. A client is admitted to a drug rehabilitation program. He appears thin with scattered lesions where he has been picking at his skin and shows evidence of severe tooth decay but is very talkative and has a rapid, irregular heartbeat. Based on these signs and symptoms, which of the following is most likely his drug of choice?

    1. cocaine
    2. methamphetamine
    3. marijuana
    4. LSD

23. A 4-year-old child with autism spectrum disorder has verbal skills but interacts poorly. The child says "bunny" and reaches for a stuffed animal that is on a shelf. Which of the following is the best example of incidental teaching?

    1. The nurse asks, "What color is the bunny?" and waits for a response before giving the child the toy.
    2. The nurse states, "That's right! That is a bunny" and gives the child the toy.
    3. The nurse gives the child the toy without comment.
    4. The nurse states, "Before you get the bunny, you need to answer some questions."

24. A 7-year-old child with special needs has difficulty learning activities that require more than one step. Which of the following approaches is likely to be the most effective?

    1. having the child master step one before progressing to step two
    2. coaching and assisting the child through each step sequentially
    3. providing posters with sequential pictures
    4. back chaining

25. A client is scheduled to undergo a cholecystectomy. Which of the following is a required element of informed consent?

    1. duration of operation
    2. names of surgical staff
    3. risks and benefits
    4. insurance coverage

26. A woman comes to the emergency department after being badly beaten. She is shaking and appears very frightened. Which of the following is the first question the nurse should ask?

1. "Who did this to you?"
2. "Is the person who did this to you present here in the hospital?"
3. "Have you called the police?"
4. "Do you want information about women's shelters?"

27. A female client complains of sudden onset of chest and abdominal "tightness" and pressure with pain in the neck and jaw. The client feels fatigued and nauseated. She appears pale and dyspneic, and her skin is cold and clammy. Which of the following diagnostic tests does the nurse anticipate will be completed initially?

1. electrocardiogram
2. bronchoscopy
3. echocardiogram
4. complete blood count

28. A client in the mental health unit tells the nurse, "I drink too much because my job is so stressful and because I need to relax." This is an example of which type of defense mechanism?

1. suppression
2. repression
3. rationalization
4. denial

29. The nurse does an admission interview with a Native American client. The client does not make eye contact and remains silent for extended periods of time and withdraws when the nurse reaches out to touch the client's hand when reassuring her about her treatment. Which of the following is the most likely reason for the client's behavior?

1. the client is frightened
2. the client is dishonest
3. the client is exhibiting cultural traits
4. the client speaks little English

30. A client tells the nurse that she has always hated her mother, who left the client behind with her abusive father when the parents divorced. The mother has been trying to reestablish a relationship with the client, who is now 23 years old, but the client remains uncertain and angry. Which spiritual need is the client grappling with?

1. love
2. faith
3. hope
4. forgiveness

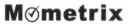

31. A client with Alzheimer's disease has repeatedly gotten out the front door at night and run away. Which of the following suggestions may be helpful to a caregiver? Select all that apply.

1. hang a curtain over the doorway
2. place a latch at the top or bottom of the door
3. lock the client into her bedroom
4. place a motion sensor with a loud alarm on the client's bedroom door
5. place bed restraints on the client

32. Which of the following client actions most indicate the potential for assaultive behavior? Select all that apply.

1. passive-aggressive behavior
2. avoidance of eye contact
3. verbal threats
4. anger disproportionate to situation
5. withdrawal

33. A client recently diagnosed with colon cancer becomes furious when the nurse gives her an injection, shouting, "You hurt me, you idiot! You are so incompetent!" Which of the following is the most likely reason for the outburst?

1. the nurse is incompetent
2. the client is in the anger stage of the grief response
3. the client is in the denial stage of the grief response
4. the client has a low pain tolerance

34. A client with dementia says to the nurse, "I'm going to the movies now. I always go to the movies on Thanksgiving evening. I hope it doesn't snow." Which is the most appropriate response?

1. "It's not Thanksgiving."
2. "What a lovely tradition! I love movies."
3. "Today is July 2. It's almost lunch time but after that you can watch a movie on TV."
4. "It's snowing, so this is not a good time to go to the movies."

35. A client with terminal cancer states she is not afraid of death but is afraid of the process of dying. Which of the following is the best response?

1. "What aspects of the dying process are you most concerned about?"
2. "Those are normal feelings."
3. "What can I do to help?"
4. "I'm so sorry."

36. A client has experienced repeated panic attacks and at a visit to a clinic periodically snaps a rubber band against his wrist. Which of the following is the most likely reason for this action?

1. the client has a nervous habit
2. the client is practicing self-injurious behavior
3. the client is trying to get attention
4. the client is practicing thought-stopping

6

37. What type of initial nursing response is the most effective for a woman undergoing a traumatic stress crisis after being raped?

1. encourage the client to express feelings about the trauma
2. encourage the client to talk about and describe the rape
3. teach the client relaxation techniques
4. tell the client about resources for rape victims

38. Which of the following are examples of normalization for pediatric clients? Select all that apply.

1. painting children's rooms in bright colors
2. providing a play area
3. allowing siblings to visit
4. facilitating doll reenactment play
5. serving meals on trays in children's rooms

39. A client in the mental health unit has a panic-level anxiety attack and has become immobile and mute and is not processing environmental stimuli. Which of the following actions is the best nursing response?

1. attempt to distract the client through music or conversation
2. remain with the client and speak in a calm, reassuring voice
3. remind the client that the anxiety will pass
4. encourage the client to use self-hypnosis techniques

40. A schizophrenic client has frequent hallucinations and is becoming increasingly withdrawn. Which of the following are appropriate interventions for hallucinations? Select all that apply.

1. communicate frequently with the client to help present reality
2. use distracting techniques
3. ask client to describe the hallucinations
4. encourage client to participate in reality-based activities, such as playing cards
5. tell client to ignore the hallucinations

41. Which of the following is the primary risk factor for cervical cancer?

1. smoking
2. chlamydia infection
3. family history of cervical cancer
4. human papillomavirus (HPV)

42. A 36-year-old woman who smokes 2 packs of cigarettes daily seeks advice about contraception. Which of the following contraceptive methods should she avoid? Select all that apply.

1. vaginal ring
2. combined hormone pills
3. intrauterine device
4. progestogen-only pill
5. all contraceptives except condoms and diaphragms

43. A client with asthma is to be discharged and must take nebulizer treatments at home. Which of the following is the best method to ensure that the client understands how to use and clean the equipment after the nurse completes a demonstration?

1. provide the client with written instructions
2. provide the client with a telephone number to call if questions arise
3. ask the client if he has any questions
4. ask the client to do a return demonstration

44. When conducting a physical examination of a 62-year-old female, the nurse notes nodules on the dorsolateral aspects of the distal interphalangeal joints (Heberden's nodes) of the right hand. Which of the following diseases does this finding suggest?

1. acute tenosynovitis
2. gout
3. rheumatoid arthritis
4. osteoarthritis

45. A mother brings her toddler to a well-baby clinic. The child is fair, and his skin is yellow-tinged, especially evident on the nose and the palms of the hands and feet; however, the sclera is white. Which of the following does the nurse anticipate should be initially assessed?

1. liver function tests
2. diet
3. blood count
4. electrolytes

46. Fetal heart tones are usually first heard with a fetoscope at what week of gestation?
Record your answer using a whole number.

47. A new mother who is Hispanic brings her one-month-old infant for a well-baby exam and reports that she is adding yams, pureed beans, and sugar to the child's formula and has enlarged the nipple to accommodate the thickened formula. Which of the following is the most likely reason for this practice?

1. the mother is following a cultural practice
2. the mother is uneducated about infant care
3. the mother cannot afford to purchase adequate amounts of formula
4. the mother is negligent

48. When taking an adult client's blood pressure, the lower border of the cuff should be how far above the antecubital crease?

1. 1 cm
2. 5 cm
3. 2.5 cm
4. 7.5 cm

49. The mother of a 6-month-old child reports that she has a very good baby who is very quiet and sleeps well. The nurse notes that when the phone rings across the room, the child continues to look at the mother. Which of the following should the nurse suspect?

1. the child has a hearing deficit
2. the child is anxious
3. the child has cognitive impairment
4. the child is exhibiting normal behavior for age

8

50. A client complains of blurred vision, fatigue, loss of appetite, weight loss, increased thirst, and frequent urination. Which of the following laboratory assessments is most indicated?

1. blood glucose and HbA1c
2. serum and urine osmolality
3. complete blood count
4. urinalysis

51. Which of the following laboratory findings are consistent with hypernatremia?

1. increased serum sodium and decreased urine sodium
2. increased serum sodium and decreased urine osmolality
3. increased serum sodium and increased urine sodium
4. increased serum sodium and decreased urine specific gravity

52. The mother of a 20-month-old child reports that another toddler in daycare developed a fever 7 days previously while in contact with the other children and subsequently was diagnosed with roseola. The mother is concerned that her child will develop roseola. What information should the nurse provide to the mother? Select all that apply.

1. roseola is contagious with onset of rash
2. the incubation period for roseola is 9 to 10 days
3. roseola is contagious with onset of fever
4. the incubation period for roseola is 3 to 6 days
5. roseola is contagious 2 days prior to onset of fever

53. A client has a large pressure sore on the coccygeal area. The pressure sore is draining large amounts of seropurulent discharge. Which of the following is the most appropriate choice for dressing material?

1. alginate
2. hydrocolloid
3. hydrogel
4. transparent film

54. A client experiences a severe generalized tonic-clonic seizure while in bed in supine position with one side rail down. Which of the following actions by the nurse are correct? Select all that apply.

1. insert a padded tongue blade between the client's teeth
2. turn client to the side-lying position
3. elevate and pad side rails
4. leave side rail down and stand on open side to restrain client if needed
5. restrain patient physically throughout the seizure

55. A home care client has been having an Unna boot replaced every 7 days, but at a home visit the nurse finds the patient cannot ambulate because of an injury to the opposite leg. Which of the following actions is most correct at this time?

1. the Unna boot should be discontinued and the leg left open
2. the Unna boot should be changed as scheduled
3. the Unna boot should be discontinued and replaced with a short stretch wrap (such as Comprilan®)
4. the Unna boot should be discontinued and another form of compression used

56. Place the following metric weight measures in the correct position in the table below.

      I. gram
      II. decigram
      III. dekagram
      IV. hectogram

Milligram	Centigram	(1)	(2)	(3)	(4)	Kilogram

      1. ____
      2. ____
      3. ____
      4. ____

57. A client has a colostomy in the following anatomic position (see diagram). When teaching the patient about colostomy care, which of the following information should the nurse include? Select all that apply.

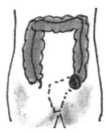

      1. "You should expect to have a bowel movement every day."
      2. "You may be able to regulate your bowel movements with diet or irrigations."
      3. "Your stool may be soft to solid."
      4. "There are different types of colostomy appliances available."
      5. "Your stool will probably be semi-liquid."

58. A 68-year-old client recently had a hip replacement for which she is receiving opioid analgesia. The patient refused dinner and exhibited sudden onset of weakness and confusion. During the assessment of the client, the nurse asks the client to show her teeth.

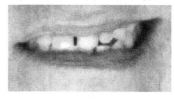

Based on the client's response (see photo), which of the following does the nurse expect is *most* likely the cause of the client's symptoms?

      1. over-medication
      2. hypoglycemia
      3. stroke
      4. delirium

59. The nurse is completing a physical examination of a client and evaluating the client for peripheral arterial and venous insufficiency. Which of the following findings are consistent with peripheral arterial insufficiency? Select all that apply.

1. brownish discoloration appears about the ankles and anterior tibial area
2. foot exhibits rubor on dependency and pallor on elevation
3. ulcers are evident on end of great toe and heel
4. peripheral edema is marked
5. ulcers are superficial and irregular, often on medial or lateral malleolus

60. A client has been recovering well from a knee replacement but has sudden onset of restlessness and anxiety and complains of chest pain, shortness of breath, and cough with frothy blood-tinged sputum. The client's pulse is 110 and temperature 101.2°F/38.4°C. The nurse notes rales in the right lung and tachypnea. Based on these findings, which of the following complications is most likely?

1. pulmonary embolism
2. atelectasis
3. pneumonia
4. pneumothorax

61. A client is recovering from abdominal surgery after a gunshot wound. When the nurse sees increased sanguineous drainage and changes the dressing, the nurse notes that the midline abdominal incision is dehiscing and a loop of the intestine has eviscerated through the lower third of the wound. While the client is awaiting transfer to surgery for repair, which of the following interventions should the nurse carry out? Select all that apply.

1. wearing sterile gloves, attempt to reinsert the viscera through the open wound
2. cover the viscera with a dry sterile dressing
3. cover the viscera with a normal saline–soaked sterile dressing
4. place the client in low Fowler's position with knees slightly flexed
5. place the client in Trendelenburg position

62. A 70-year-old female states that she has difficulty falling asleep and sleeps poorly, often lying awake much of the night. The nurse should anticipate which of the following as the initial intervention?

1. assessment of sleep patterns
2. nocturnal polysomnogram
3. prescription for hypnotic
4. dietary modifications

63. The nurse is interviewing a 56-year-old male with obstructive sleep apnea (OSA) for which he has been prescribed a CPAP machine for use during sleep. The client yawns frequently during the interview. Which of the following statements by the client indicates a need for further education about OSA and CPAP?

1. "I use only distilled water for humidification."
2. "I try to use the CPAP most nights."
3. "I wash the mask and tubing with soap and water and rinse with water and vinegar."
4. "I think the nasal mask is better than the orofacial mask."

64. A 26-year-old client is going to use continuous ambulatory peritoneal dialysis (CAPD) after discharge from the hospital. Which of the following should the nurse include in teaching about CAPD? Select all that apply.

1. "You will instill about 2 liters of fluid over 10 to 15 minutes."
2. "Clamp the tubing and maintain a dwell time of about 30 minutes."
3. "Unclamp the tubing and drain for about 20 minutes."
4. "Immerse the dialysate bag in warm water to increase temperature."
5. "You will instill about 2 liters of fluid over 3 to 5 hours."

65. A 5-year-old child is undergoing chemotherapy for acute lymphocytic leukemia (ALL). The child has weekly blood tests to monitor status. Which of the following abnormalities of the blood are of most concern during treatment for leukemia?

1. thrombocytopenia and neutropenia
2. thrombocytosis and neutropenia
3. thrombocytosis and neutrocytosis
4. thrombocytopenia and neutrocytosis

66. A 35-year-old woman is recovering from a thyroidectomy for Hashimoto's thyroiditis. The client complains that she is experiencing a tingling sensation about her mouth and fingers and muscle cramps in her legs. Which of the following complications is most likely the cause of these symptoms?

1. hypocalcemia
2. hypercalcemia
3. hypermagnesemia
4. hypomagnesemia

67. According to USDA dietary guidelines (see diagram), which of the following meals most corresponds to dietary recommendations?

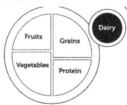

1. one apple, 1 cup carrots, 1 cup long-grain white rice, 4 ounces poached salmon, and ½ cup sweetened yogurt
2. one cup canned fruit cocktail, 1 cup corn, 1 cup long-grain white rice, 4 ounces fried breaded fish sticks, and 8 ounces of wine
3. one cup steamed kale, one medium baked potato with butter and sour cream, 6 ounces rib-eye steak, and 1 cup of coffee
4. one-half banana, 1 cup broccoli, ½ cup quinoa, 3 ounces roasted turkey, and 8 ounces of 1% milk

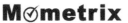

68. The mother of an 11-year-old boy asks the nurse what type of anticipatory guidance she should provide for her son. Which of the following are age-appropriate topics the nurse should suggest for a child of this age? Select all that apply.

1. what to expect in terms of physical development and secondary sexual characteristics
2. responsibilities of sexual behavior, including abstinence and birth control
3. peer group pressures, including gangs, alcohol, and tobacco use
4. future goals and plans
5. dating and relationship issues

69. A neonate has hyperbilirubinemia and jaundice, and the physician has prescribed phototherapy, which the nurse is about to administer.

I. Place a protective mask over the child's eyes.
II. Adjust light source to 15 to 20 cm above child.
III. Turn on lights.
IV. Remove all clothes except diaper.

Place the actions listed above (Roman numerals) in order, beginning with the first action.

1. (First action)
2. (Second action)
3. (Third action)
4. (Fourth action)

70. A client comes to a clinic with a severe cough and fever, but all of the exam rooms are full when the client arrives. Which of the following is the best action for the nurse to take?

1. tell the client to reschedule an appointment for a less busy hour
2. ask the client to wait outside until an exam room becomes available
3. provide the client a facemask and seat her in the waiting area with other clients
4. provide the client a facemask and seat the client in a separate area as far as possible from other clients

71. A pregnant woman at 21 weeks gestation has severe pre-eclampsia with BP of 170/120 and proteinuria of 6 g in 24 hours. What treatment does the nurse anticipate is initially indicated?

1. bedrest only
2. phenytoin
3. magnesium sulfate
4. antihypertensive, such as hydralazine

72. A full-term pregnant woman experienced premature rupture of the membranes 24 hours earlier but has not gone into labor. Which of the following does the nurse anticipate?

1. labor will be induced
2. client is at increased risk of hemorrhage
3. client will undergo Caesarean
4. labor will be induced if the patient does not go into labor within 48 hours

13

73. A patient had a bowel resection and has been reluctant to take deep breaths and cough because of discomfort. Which of the following interventions is most indicated initially to prevent atelectasis?

1. regular use of incentive spirometer
2. nebulizer treatments with albuterol
3. IPPB treatments
4. prophylactic antibiotics

74. A client has had a pacemaker inserted recently but complains that he is experiencing heart palpitations and generalized weakness and that he has slight pain in the chest and jaw. On examination, the nurse notes that the client appears quite anxious, and the nurse observes pulsations in the neck and abdomen. Which of the following is the most likely cause of these findings?

1. pacemaker wiring has become dislodged
2. infection
3. coronary artery occlusion
4. pacemaker syndrome

75. A client on cardiac monitoring has dislodged his leads 6 times in a 4-hour period, setting off alarms. Each time, he makes a different excuse, but the nurse suspects the dislodgements are purposeful because the client attempts to delay the nurse's leaving after each episode. Which of the following is the most appropriate response?

1. "I can see that you are doing this on purpose."
2. "These constant alarms are disturbing to other patients."
3. "Why are you disconnecting your leads?"
4. "Let's talk about the reason for monitoring and what we can learn from it."

76. Which of the following should never be delegated to unlicensed assistive personnel?

1. monitoring and controlling blood therapy
2. bathing patient
3. ambulating patient
4. monitoring urinary output

77. Prior to irrigating a nasogastric (NG) tube, the nurse gently aspirates fluid and then measures the pH of the aspirate with color-coded pH paper. Which of the following pH values is consistent with gastric fluid?

1. 6
2. 5
3. 4.4
4. 3.8

78. A client has had three recent bouts of cystitis and now has urinary frequency and burning, chills, fever of 102°F/38.9°C, abdominal pain, and bilateral flank pain. Which of the following diagnostic tests does the nurse expect the physician to order initially?

1. complete blood count
2. urinalysis and urine culture and sensitivities
3. kidney function tests
4. cystoscopy

79. A client is receiving radiotherapy to the abdominal area and has developed chronic diarrhea. Which of the following should the nurse include when teaching the client ways to manage the diarrhea? Select all that apply.

1. "It's important to drink 8 to 12 glasses of clear fluids each day."
2. "It's better to eat 5 or 6 small meals than 3 large meals."
3. "Try to increase the fiber in your diet."
4. "You can try the BRAT diet (banana, rice, applesauce, and toast)."
5. "Drinking milk and eating ice cream may soothe your stomach."

80. A client has been on a weight-loss program. Her waist measures 28 inches and hips 40 inches. What is her waist-to-hip ratio? *Record your answer using a decimal number.*

81. The nurse is planning to empty a Jackson-Pratt drainage device for a client following a mastectomy. Before emptying the bulb, the nurse notes a number of large clots in the tubing. Which of the following is the most appropriate response?

1. leave the clots undisturbed
2. notify the physician that the device needs to be changed
3. irrigate the tubing with normal saline
4. milk the tubing before emptying the device

82. The nurse is discussing the use of a condom with a sexually active 17-year-old male client being treated for gonorrhea. Which of the following information should the nurse include? Select all that apply.

1. use a condom every time for every sexual encounter
2. use natural membrane condoms, which provide better protection than latex
3. use only water-based lubricants
4. hold the condom in place when withdrawing the penis after ejaculation
5. apply the condom so it fits snugly against the glans of the penis

83. A client is treated in the emergency department for second-degree burns after falling asleep while sunbathing. The client states she sunbathes 8 to 10 hours every week to maintain a tan. Which of the following advice is most important to share with the client? Select all that apply.

1. excessive exposure to the sun increases the risk of skin cancer
2. the client should limit tanning to 2 to 3 hours at a time
3. self-tanners are available that do not require sun exposure
4. there is no value in exposing the skin to the sun
5. sunscreen should be applied for prolonged exposure to the sun

84. A client with diabetes has been advised by the physician to do strength training twice a week and to engage in aerobic activities. The client has indicated an interest in walking, which is a moderate aerobic exercise. How many minutes per week should the client be advised to walk to meet current exercise guidelines? Record your answer using a whole number.

_____ minutes.

85. The nurse must teach a female client to carry out clean intermittent catheterization (CIC). The steps to the procedure (in Roman numerals) include:

   I. locate meatus (by touch or with mirror)
   II. insert catheter and hold in place until urine stops draining
   III. spread labia and cleanse area with soap and water
   IV. lubricate catheter (with water soluble lubricant)

Place the steps in Roman numerals the correct order.

   1. (Step 1) _____
   2. (Step 2) _____
   3. (Step 3) _____
   4. (Step 4) _____

86. The nurse is a member of a team in which two members have an escalating personal conflict that is affecting team morale and functioning. Which of the following initial responses is most appropriate?

   1. tell the two members they are acting childishly
   2. report the two members to the unit supervisor
   3. express concern and offer to mediate
   4. ignore the situation as much as possible

87. Which of the following is the most effective scale for assessing pain in a 6-year-old child?

   1. Wong-Baker FACES pain scale
   2. 0-10 numeric pain intensity scale
   3. PAINAD scale
   4. CRIES scale

88. A client has pancreatic cancer, stage 4, and is taking high doses of morphine to control severe pain. Which statement by the client's spouse and caregiver suggests a need for education?

   1. "The morphine doesn't seem to be working as well now."
   2. "I think death will be a relief for both of us."
   3. "This experience has shaken my belief in God."
   4. "I know all this morphine is making her a drug addict."

89. A female client's CBC showed the following results:

Test	Result
WBC	4.1 (10^3/µL)
RBC	4.38 (10^6/µL)
Hemoglobin	13.8 (g/dL)
Hematocrit	42 (%)
Platelet count	116 (10^3/µL)

Which of the tests are outside of the normal range?

   1. hemoglobin and hematocrit
   2. all tests are outside of normal range.
   3. platelet count and WBC
   4. platelet count and RBC

90. A client has had a stroke in the right hemisphere and has pronounced weakness on the left side and expressive aphasia. The nurse notes that the client has some dysphagia and is concerned that the client may aspirate. The nurse plans to ask the doctor about a referral to have the client's swallowing evaluated. The most appropriate referral is to which healthcare professional?

    1. speech and language therapist
    2. occupational therapist
    3. physical therapist
    4. EENT specialist

91. When inserting a nasogastric feeding tube, the nurse pauses after inserting about 25 cm of tubing, listens at the distal end of the tubing, and hears air exchange. Which of the following is the most appropriate response?

    1. continue to insert tube but withdraw if coughing becomes excessive
    2. continue to slowly insert tube while patient swallows sips of water
    3. pull the tube back approximately 10 cm and then reinsert
    4. remove the tube and start the procedure again

92. A nurse is assessing a client with suspected diabetes mellitus, type 1. Which of the following signs and symptoms are consistent with this diagnosis? Select all that apply.

    1. polyuria, polydipsia, and polyphagia
    2. Kussmaul breathing
    3. recent weight gain
    4. weakness, fatigue
    5. blurred vision

93. The nurse must move a patient who is lying supine onto the side of the bed in preparation for transfer to a wheelchair. The steps to this procedure include the following:

    I. roll client onto side, facing nurse
    II. place one hand under shoulders and the other over the hips
    III. raise head of bed to 30°
    IV. pivot the client into a sitting position

Place the steps (in Roman numerals) into the correct order:

    1. (First) _____
    2. (Second) _____
    3. (Third) _____
    4. (Fourth) _____

94. A client who is receiving total parenteral nutrition (TPN) has weakness and dizziness. The client is diaphoretic, pale, and lethargic, as well as increasingly confused. Which of the following laboratory tests is most indicated?

    1. serum albumin
    2. serum glucose
    3. electrolytes
    4. triglyceride level

95. A client in the cardiac care unit has been very upset since two other clients in the unit died and tells the nurse, "Everyone dies here. I don't know why you are bothering treating me." Which of the following is the most therapeutic response?

1. "You are worried that you're going to die."
2. "You are recovering well, so you don't need to worry."
3. "The other clients were much sicker than you are."
4. "You should discuss your concerns with your doctor."

96. The nurse is floated to the oncology unit but has not had previous experience administering IV chemotherapy, which the nurse must administer to two clients. Which of the following is the most appropriate response?

1. research the drugs and correct administration prior to giving them
2. ask one of the other nurses to assist with administration
3. discuss the lack of experience with the unit supervisor
4. refuse to administer the chemotherapy

97. An 8-year-old child is brought to the emergency department with her tongue partially severed. The parents state that the child accidentally bit her tongue. The child is crying and appears frightened and withdrawn. Which of the following actions is most appropriate?

1. report the incident to Child Protective Services
2. accept the parents' report of the accident
3. ask the child what really happened
4. tell the parents the injury could not be accidental

98. The nurse observed another nurse remove a hydrocodone tablet from a client's medicine drawer and then swallow the tablet when it appeared no one was looking. Which of the following is the most appropriate response?

1. immediately report the incident to a direct supervisor
2. immediately confront the nurse
3. report the incident to the police
4. report the incident to the client's physician

99. A 38-year-old client with rheumatoid arthritis tells the nurse that she is having increasing difficulty dressing herself and managing activities of daily living at home because of her disabilities. Which referral may be most effective?

1. physical therapist
2. occupational therapist
3. housekeeping service
4. home health agency

100. The nurse is using motivational interviewing with a client who is addicted to heroin, to change behaviors. Which of the following are important elements of motivational interviewing? Select all that apply.

1. express empathy instead of criticism
2. focus on client's weaknesses
3. avoid confrontation
4. listen instead of giving advice
5. actively oppose client resistance

101. A client is exhibiting local manifestation of inflammation about a wound. Which of the following are characteristic of inflammation? Select all that apply.

1. pain/tenderness
2. edema
3. rubor
4. purulent discharge
5. dehiscence

102. The nurse has transported a mother and newborn by wheelchair to the car when the mother is being discharged in order to verify that the parents have a car seat. Which of the following is the most appropriate method of ensuring correct use?

1. check installation, question parents, and observe
2. ask parents if they have installed the car seat properly and know use
3. observe the parents placing the newborn in the car seat
4. tell the parents to be sure to read literature about car seats

103. A client tells the nurse that his physician has advised him to take over-the-counter (OTC) anti-inflammatory drugs to control the discomfort of osteoarthritis. The client asks the nurse what drugs to consider. Which of the following medications should the nurse advise the client are OTC anti-inflammatory drugs? Select all that apply.

1. NSAIDs
2. corticosteroids
3. acetaminophen
4. salicylates

104. A client with a large pressure sore is suffering from malnutrition and has had little protein in her diet. What effect does inadequate protein intake have on wound healing?

1. no or minimal effect
2. inhibits phagocytosis of white blood cells
3. slows healing process because of lack of amino acids
4. causes vasoconstriction that impairs circulation

105. A client is admitted to the hospital from a board-and-care facility with a coccygeal pressure sore that is 5 × 8 cm in size and involves partial thickness loss of dermis and red/pink wound surface without slough. Based on these observations, what stage is the pressure ulcer?

1. stage I
2. stage II
3. stage III
4. stage IV

106. When examining a client's abdomen, in which areas of the abdomen would the nurse expect to locate the following abdominal structures?

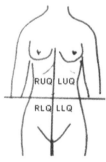

      I. spleen
      II. part of descending colon
      III. liver and gallbladder
      IV. cecum and appendix

Place the Roman numerals representing the abdominal structures in the correct quadrant:
    1. RUQ:
    2. LUQ:
    3. RLQ:
    4. LLQ:

107. A client receiving total parenteral nutrition (TPN) must receive 2 grams of protein per kilogram of body weight per day. The patient weighs 136.4 lb. How many total grams of protein should the client receive each day? Record your answer using a whole number.

      _____ grams

108. On admission to the hospital for surgery, a client reports being allergic to kiwi fruit, bananas, and avocados. Based on these allergies, for which other allergy is the client especially at risk?
    1. adhesive
    2. bee sting
    3. pineapples
    4. latex

109. Which of the following are examples of autoimmune disorders? Select all that apply.
    1. Guillain-Barré syndrome
    2. diabetes mellitus, type 1
    3. rheumatoid arthritis
    4. Hashimoto thyroiditis
    5. osteoarthritis
    6. diabetes mellitus, type 2

110. The nurse notes that a portable electrocardiogram machine that is in frequent use has a frayed electrical cord. Which of the following is the most appropriate initial response?
    1. place tape around the frayed section of cord
    2. tape a "beware frayed cord" notice to the machine
    3. immediately remove the machine from service
    4. notify the unit supervisor that the machine needs repair

111. The nurse is working in the emergency department when a multi-car accident occurs on a nearby interstate highway, resulting in many casualties. The following injured people are the first to arrive:

> I. 64-year-old woman, alert and responsive, with large laceration on the head
> II. 16-year-old male with chest injury in respiratory distress and severe pain
> III. 28-year old male with multiple contusions and fractured right arm
> IV. very agitated, hallucinating, and confused middle-aged male with unknown injuries but reeking of alcohol

If carrying out triage and considering the severity of injury, in which order (indicating with Roman numeral) should the clients be treated?

- (First) _____
- (Second) _____
- (Third) _____
- (Fourth) _____

112. A client with osteomyelitis of the right tibia that has cultured positive for *Staphylococcus aureus* is to be discharged home with dressing changes done daily by nurses from a home health agency. When teaching family members about infection control, which of the following is the most important point to stress?

1. limiting contact with others
2. sterilizing environmental surfaces
3. wearing gowns and gloves for all contact with client
4. handwashing

113. If a nurse must move a heavy cart full of supplies, which of the following techniques uses the best body mechanics?

1. push the cart from behind with both hands, keeping head up and back straight.
2. pull the cart from ahead with one hand, leaning forward slightly.
3. push the cart from behind, pushing against it with the shoulders.
4. pull the cart from ahead with one hand, keeping head up and back straight.

114. The nurse is assisting a 19-year-old client who is not allowed weight bearing on the left foot with crutch walking, and the client states he wants to keep pace with his friends when they are walking. Which of the following crutch gaits requires the most energy but allows the fastest gait?

1. 4-point alternate
2. swing-through
3. swing-to
4. 2-point alternate

115. A client who recently tripped and fell is to begin using a rolling walker with wheels in the front only. What is the best method to properly adjust the walker to the correct height for the client?

1. try different adjustments until one seems comfortable for the client.
2. measure the distance from midway between elbow and wrist and adjust walker to that eight.
3. adjust the height so that the client can comfortably lean forward and bear weight onto walker.
4. measure distance from wrist to floor and adjust walker to that height.

116. The sharps containers in the clients' hospital rooms contain the following symbol:

What does this symbol signify?
1. poison
2. danger
3. biohazard
4. sharps

117. If the nurse has made a medication error, giving the wrong client a dosage of antacid, which of the following is the appropriate action?
1. no action is required as antacids are harmless
2. notify the physician, document the medication given, and file an incident report
3. notify the physician only
4. ask the physician for a retroactive order for an antacid

118. If a client who had abdominal surgery the previous day experiences evisceration and the nurse finds intestines protruding from the wound, what initial step should the nurse take to protect the wound?
1. cover with saline soaked sterile dressings
2. cover with a dry sterile dressing
3. cover the wound with plastic
4. leave the wound exposed to air

119. The nurse is working in a hospital unit when a tornado levels a large shopping mall near the hospital, resulting in mass casualties. The hospital is on alert and has advised staff that hospital beds must be freed for incoming injured. What immediate action should the nurse take?
1. wait for further directions
2. inform current clients they will probably be discharged
3. make a list of noncritical clients who might be safely discharged
4. start calling physicians to ask if their clients can be discharged

120. If a long-time user of opioids is administered naloxone (Narcan) for an opioid overdose, which of the following may occur as a result of the reversal agent?
1. Parkinsonian-like tremors
2. confusion and disorientation
3. hyperthermia
4. withdrawal and seizures

Answer Key and Explanations for Test #1

1. 2: Because penicillin may cause an anaphylactic reaction, especially in someone who has previously has a milder reaction, the correct action is to hold the drug and notify the prescribing physician that the client may have had a drug reaction so that the physician can order a skin test or an alternate antibiotic. Common adverse effects of penicillin include rash, hives, itching, and edema of face, lips, and/or tongue. Anaphylactic reactions usually occur within 60 minutes of contact with the causative agent.

2. 3: Fresh frozen plasma replaces plasma but does not contain red blood cells or platelets. It does, however, contain most coagulation factors and complement, so it is the blood product of choice for disorders in which coagulation factors are needed. **Whole blood** is rarely used but replaces both red blood cells and plasma. **Irradiated red blood cells** are used to replace red blood cells in those who are immunocompromised. **Platelets** are used for those with thrombocytopenia.

3. 3: Even though the client indicated he might want the medication at a later time, the medication must be disposed of following facility protocol with two witnesses, both of whom are licensed to dispense medications and directly observe the disposal and sign a document verifying the disposal. A medication removed from a medicine cart may not be placed back into the cart, and drugs cannot be left at a client's bedside or kept in an unsecure location, such as a tray, for later administration.

4. Seventy-five (75) drops per minute. In order to complete the calculation, the time needs to be converted to minutes. Three hours and 20 minutes equals 200 minutes. Then, the flow rate (mL per minute) is calculated by dividing the total volume by the minutes: 1000 mL/200 minutes equals 5 mL per minute. Since there are 15 drops per mL and 5 mL per minute, the flow rate is 15 X 5 equals 75 drops per minute.

5. 1: While protocols may vary slightly, generally those receiving brachytherapy are restricted to a private room during the duration of therapy. Women who are pregnant and children under age 18 may not visit, and visitors are limited to no more than 2 hours visit per day. Visitors must remain at least 6 feet away from the client during visits. Nurses must limit time in the room to that necessary for essential care. Housekeeping staff should be accompanied by a nurse if entering the room is necessary.

6. 2: Once a sterile field is contaminated, everything within the field is also considered contaminated, so the nurse must discard the sterile field and gauze pads and start over with new supplies. When establishing a sterile field, the nurse must ensure that the area under the sterile field is clean and dry, as moisture will contaminate the field. The nurse uses clean gloves to remove the old dressing and bare hands or new clean gloves to open the sterile field and gauze packages but dons sterile gloves to apply new dressings.

7. 12 mL: The first calculation is to determine the amount of drug per milligram: 100/10 = 10 mg per mL. Then, the total dose is divided by the dose per mL: 120/10 = 12 mL. The calculation can also be done by a simple algebraic formula:

$100/10 = 120/x$
$100x = 1200$
$x = 12$

23

8. 3: The most common treatment for both strains (pulled muscles) and sprains (joint damage) is RICE therapy. **Rest** avoids further injury and lets the tissue begin to heal. **Ice/cold compresses** (15–20 minutes per hour for 24 to 48 hours) helps to reduce edema. **Compression** (such as with Ace bandages) helps to reduce edema and prevent further swelling. **Elevation** (above the heart) helps to decrease edema by increasing drainage. RICE is usually sufficient for first-degree sprains, but second- or third-degree sprains may require splinting to support the joint.

9. 4: Regardless of experience or position, every nurse is responsible for the safety and welfare of clients, so the nurse should immediately tell the team leader that the irrigating syringe was contaminated and offer to retrieve new sterile supplies. Accidents happen, and one incident does not necessarily mean the team leader is negligent. This is a matter for a supervisor only if the team leader ignores the nurse and continues with the irrigation using a contaminated syringe, putting the client at increased risk of infection.

10. 2: The AED kit contains cutting shears so that the nurse can quickly expose the chest. The nurse should use the shears to cut away bras with metal wires because the wires may cause arcing during defibrillation. Likewise, any metal piercings on the chest, such as nipple rings, should be removed. The defibrillator electrodes are placed on the right upper chest (negative) and below and lateral to the heart on the left side (positive). AEDs provide spoken messages and diagrams to guide people through the process.

11. 15 mg: In this case, calculation involves only multiplying the number of kilograms of weight (60) times the milligrams per kilogram (0.5). Thus, 60 X 0.5 = 30 mg per 24 hours. Since the drug is to be given in two equal doses (30/2), each dose is 15 mg.

12. 3: While digoxin is used to slow the heart rate, digoxin toxicity may result in either tachycardia or bradycardia as well as almost any type of dysrhythmia. Central nervous system symptoms can include fatigue, headache, and confusion with convulsions with severe toxicity. Clients often complain of GI upsets, including lack of appetite, diarrhea, nausea, and vomiting. They may also report visual disturbances, such as halo vision, colored vision, and flickering lights. The medication should be stopped immediately and cardiac monitoring started with symptoms treated as necessary.

13. 1, 3, 4, and 5: Drug compliance is especially important for seizure disorders, and since phenytoin is usually given once or twice daily, the client should establish a routine of taking the drug at the same times each day. Phenytoin may cause gingival hyperplasia, so careful dental care and routine dental evaluations are necessary. Long-term use of phenytoin may also cause osteoporosis, so people should take vitamin D prophylactically and exercise regularly as well as having periodic evaluations of osteoporosis to determine if other medications are necessary.

14. 1: Loop diuretics, such as furosemide, block chloride and sodium resorption in the ascending limb of the loop of Henle, bringing about rapid diuresis but with major electrolyte disturbance, especially hypokalemia and hyponatremia and to a lesser degree hypocalcemia. Hypokalemia is of most importance because it can result in dysrhythmias with ECG abnormalities, hypotension, lethargy, weakness, nausea and vomiting, paresthesias, muscle cramping, and tetany. Normal values are 3.5 to 5.5 mEq/L. Potassium supplementation is often given routinely with loop diuretics.

15. 1, 2, 3, and 5: A newly diagnosed client with diabetes type 1 may feel overwhelmed with information, but the nurse must ensure the client understands basic information about glucose testing and insulin administration, skin care, and dietary compliance. The client must also be taught how to respond to signs of hypoglycemia and hyperglycemia and when to call the physician. The client also needs practical information about how to store medications, where to obtain supplies, and how often to have blood tests, such as HbA1c.

16. 3: Infants are usually uncooperative with eye drops and instinctually clinch the eyes tightly to avoid them. The most appropriate method is to gently restrain the head in neutral position while the child is lying supine and place the drops at the inner canthus. When the baby opens the eyes, the fluid will flow into the eye. A caregiver, such as a parent, can assist by restraining the child's head and speaking to the child during the procedure.

17. 2: The **ventrogluteal site** is the preferred site for intramuscular injections because the muscle is deep and there is no proximity to major blood vessels or nerves, making this the safest site for injections. The **deltoid site** is commonly used for immunizations in toddlers, children, and adults, but not infants. Injections to the deltoid should be limited to 1 mL. The **dorsogluteal site** was formerly a common site, but it is close to the sciatic nerve and is currently not recommended for use. The **vastus lateralis** is also a safe site and is used for immunizations for infants.

18. 3: Piggyback units should be hung at least 6 inches higher than the primary intravenous unit. Because of the force of gravity when the piggyback unit is infusing, the flow from the primary unit stops until the piggyback unit is empty and then it starts again, so clamping the primary unit tubing is not necessary. During infusion of the piggyback unit, a backcheck valve prevents the piggyback solution from flowing up into the primary unit.

19. 1, 2, 4, and 5: The nurse should always check client identification and allergies prior to administering any medication. With IV push medication, the manufacturer's guidelines for dosage and the correct dilution should be checked because improperly diluting a medication may result in complications. Most IV push medications are administered slowly over 1 to 5 minutes, but some medications, such as adenosine, must be injected rapidly, so the recommended administration time should be adhered to, using a watch to verify time rather than approximating.

20. 3: After administration of a vaginal suppository, the woman must remain in supine position for 5 to 10 minutes to allow time for the suppository to melt and the medication to spread throughout the vagina. The suppository should be at room temperature prior to administration. If an applicator is available, it should be inserted deeply into the vagina. If inserting the suppository digitally, the finger should be inserted about 2 inches into the vagina so that the suppository rests at the cervix. The woman may want to wear a peri-pad or panty shield to contain any discharge.

21. 4: Pyridoxine (Vitamin B6) can reverse the effects of levodopa in doses exceeding 10 mg. Foods high in vitamin B6 include bran, liver, fish (salmon, cod), pork tenderloin, tahini, molasses, and hazelnuts. Levodopa should be taken with meals to minimize gastrointestinal effects, but with minimal protein at the time the medication is taken. Clients should eat proteins in small frequent amounts at other times. The client should drink at least 2 liters of fluid daily.

22. 2: Methamphetamine is a psychostimulant that can be snorted, ingested orally, smoked, or injected intravenously. While methamphetamine has similar effects to cocaine, the effect is much longer lasting and can persist up to 24 hours. Methamphetamine is often taken with alcohol to temper the anxiety that may occur, but the combination may increase blood pressure and risk of heart attack or stroke. Methamphetamine users often pick at their skin, leaving lesions that appear as severe acne, and may lose weight because of lack of appetite. "Meth mouth" with dental decay is a common sign.

23. 1: Incidental teaching uses a child's interests as teaching opportunities and motivation to respond for those with autism spectrum disorder. This type of teaching is not classroom-based. The best example is when the nurse asks, "What color is the bunny?" and waits for a correct response before giving the child the desired toy. Questions should be appropriate for the child's age and abilities. Objective questions are easier for children with autism spectrum disorder than subjective questions.

24. 4: Back chaining is an approach that teaches the last step in a process first and once that is mastered adds the next-to-the-last step, and so on until the task is mastered. For example, if teaching a child to make a peanut butter and jelly sandwich, the last step would be to place the sandwich on a plate, so the nurse would do everything except that and then ask the child to put the completed sandwich on the plate, waiting until the child masters this successfully before adding the next-to-the-last step.

25. 3: According to the American Medical Association, informed consent must include the following:

- Explanation of diagnosis
- Nature and reason for treatment or procedure
- Risks and benefits
- Alternative options (regardless of cost or insurance coverage)
- Risks and benefits of alternative options
- Risks and benefits of not having a treatment or procedure

Providing informed consent is a requirement of all states. The client should be given full and clear information prior to signing the consent form and should be encouraged to ask questions to clarify any information that is not clear.

26. 2: Because abusers often accompany victims of domestic abuse to the hospital, the first question should be "Is the person who did this to you present here in the hospital?" If the client answers affirmatively, then security should be called immediately for the client's and nurse's protection. Even if the client answers negatively, the nurse should observe carefully any interactions the client has with someone accompanying her, as she may be too frightened or too ashamed to answer truthfully.

27. 1: The initial diagnostic test should be the electrocardiogram because these symptoms are consistent with myocardial infarctions in females, who may not experience the "classic" symptoms of crushing chest pain more associated with males. Females often complain of chest or abdominal tightness and pressure and pain in the neck, jaw, shoulders, or arms rather than the chest. Some clients may complain of "indigestion" and most feel severe fatigue. Nausea, dyspnea, and cold, clammy skin are common findings.

28. 3: This is an example of **rationalization** because the client is attempting to make excuses for drinking excessively. Clients often try to find logical reasons for their actions and often blame their situations, family members, or friends for their problems. With **repression**, the client involuntarily blocks the awareness of negative feelings and experiences. **Suppression** is similar to repression, but the blocking of awareness is voluntary. **Denial** is a refusal to acknowledge that a problem exists at all.

29. 3: While all of these are possibilities, the most likely reason is simply that the client is exhibiting cultural traits common to Native Americans. Native Americans often avoid direct eye contact as a way to show respect and politeness, and they tend to be more comfortable with silence during a conversation than is typical in American culture. Native Americans also value personal space and may be uncomfortable with touch. They may feel more comfortable with folk approaches to healing rather than Western medicine and may want to combine both during treatment.

30. 4: The client is grappling with the spiritual need to forgive. Forgiveness can be very difficult—both forgiving the self and others—and clients may obsess over mistakes they or others have made. Clients may believe that forgiving someone means accepting or condoning the behavior; however, forgiving can be freeing for the client and relieve the stress associated with anger towards someone. Even if clients are unable to forgive, they may be able to make peace with what has occurred and move forward more positively.

31. 1 and 2: Disguising the doorway by hanging a curtain across it or placing a painting on the door is enough to prevent some clients with dementia from opening the door. A good way to keep clients inside is to place a latch at the top or bottom of the door as Alzheimer's clients rarely look beyond the doorknob when trying to open a door. Clients should never be locked into a room, and motion sensors with alarms are often terrifying to clients, increasing their stress and need to get away.

32. 3 and 4: While clients who are angry may exhibit passive-aggressive behavior and may avoid eye contact or stare at others, those who have the potential for assaultive behavior are usually more threatening and may make verbal threats ("I'll kill you!") or physical threats (pushing, shoving) with anger disproportionate to situation. They are often very tense and agitated, pacing and exhibiting restlessness. They often use a loud intimidating voice with shouting and obscenities. They may respond excessively to environmental stimuli and have disturbed thought processes and suspicions of others.

33. 2: The client is probably in the anger stage of the grief process (Kübler-Ross). Upon receiving bad news, many clients initially experience **denial**, although this period usually only lasts one to two weeks. Within a few hours of receiving bad news, many also begin to experience **anger**, and this anger is often directed at family members and caregivers because clients feel helpless and terrified. Many also go through a **bargaining** stage where they may begin attending religious services or seek other opinions. **Depression** may be prolonged as the client comes to grips with loss and finally reaches **acceptance**.

34. 3: As much as possible, clients with dementia should be oriented to what is true but without directly challenging them or telling them they are wrong, and the nurse should avoid humoring clients by playing along with their confused statements. In this case, telling the date (July 2) and the time (lunch time) helps to orient the client, and offering to allow the client to watch a movie responds to the client's stated desire to go a movie. If the client becomes extremely agitated at being contradicted, then the best response may be to refocus the client's attention.

35. 1: "What aspects of the dying process are you most concerned about?" is the best response because it encourages the client to express her concerns and allows the nurse to assess what can be done to alleviate those concerns. For example, many people facing death are afraid of dying in pain, and the nurse can assure that client that adequate control of pain is almost always possible. This provides a good opportunity also to discuss hospice care. Some clients may express concern about family or financial obligations. These clients may benefit from the assistance of a social worker.

36. 4: The client is probably practicing thought-stopping. This is a technique that people sometimes use to stop the intrusion of negative thoughts or anxiety. Initially, clients learn the technique by imagining something that causes them to have negative thoughts, such as the fear of being in public, and then they shout, "STOP," and attempt to redirect thoughts. Over time, they speak the word "stop" and then may substitute a silent thought. Some people use the snap of a rubber band against the skin to stop thoughts.

37. 1: While all of these things have value, clients who have been raped often find it difficult to talk about the rape itself initially but may more easily discuss their feelings—fear, anger, shame—so that is a good place to begin. Providing too much information too early, such as about relaxation techniques and resources, often serves little purpose because the client is too traumatized to process the information. Clients undergoing a traumatic stress crisis are victims of stressors over which they have no control, and this can leave them feeling overwhelmed and depressed.

38. 1, 2, and 3: Normalization is the process of providing a child with as normal an environment as possible in a facility, such as a hospital. Rooms may be painted in bright colors and play areas provided. Visiting hours are usually unrestricted, and siblings (and sometimes therapy animals) are allowed to visit. Children may eat in communal areas and be allowed more choices related to foods and sleeping hours. Planned play activities and group activities may be available for children as well. Doll reenactment is a therapeutic play technique.

39. 2: Panic attacks usually subside within 5 to 30 minutes, and the best nursing response is to stay with the client while the panic attack occurs, speaking in a calm reassuring voice even though the client in the acute stage may not be processing verbal input. Maintaining the client's safety is a primary concern because during panic attacks clients may bolt and run, even sometimes injuring themselves in the process. Quieting the environment and reducing stimuli may help reduce the client's anxiety.

40. 1, 3, and 4: The nurse should ask the client to describe hallucinations because this information is necessary to help the nurse calm the client and to determine if the client or others are at risk because of the hallucinations. The nurse should communicate frequently with the client, helping to keep the client oriented and presenting a model of reality. The nurse should also encourage the client to participate in reality-based activities, such as playing cards or badminton. Using distracting techniques is helpful when intervening for delusions but less successful with hallucinations.

41. 4: The primary risk factor for cervical cancer is a history of human papillomavirus infection. HPV comprises >100 viruses. About 40 are sexually transmitted and invade mucosal tissue, causing genital warts (condylomata). HPV infection causes changes in the mucosa, which can lead to cervical cancer. Over 99% of cervical cancers are caused by HPV, and 70% are related to HPVs 16 and 18. The HPV vaccine, Gardasil®, protects against HPVs 6 and 11 (which cause genital warts), 16 and 18 (which cause cancer). Protection is only conveyed if the female has not yet been infected with these strains.

42. 1 and 2: While most contraceptives are relatively safe for women who smoke, smokers over age 35 are usually advised to avoid combined hormone pills and vaginal rings, such as NuvaRing® (which releases both estrogen and progestogen). The women may more safely take progestogen-only pills or use an intrauterine device, intrauterine system, or diaphragm as well as implanted contraceptives and the contraceptive injection.

43. 4: While there is value in all of these approaches—written instructions, help number, questions—the best method is to ask the client to do a return demonstration. This allows the nurse to directly observe and evaluate the client's ability to carry out the needed actions. The client should be able to refer to written directions during the demonstration, but if the client requires the nurse's assistance or becomes confused, this indicates the need for further education.

44. 4: Heberden's nodes are characteristic of osteoarthritis. Other findings may include radial deviation of the distal phalanx (fingertip tilted toward the thumb) and Bouchard's nodes, nodules on the proximal interphalangeal joints. Osteoarthritis is usually caused by previous injury to joints, so it may occur on one side only, and is associated with cartilage deterioration. It is slowly progressive with symptoms usually occurring after age 60.

45. 2: Carotemia causes a yellowing of the skin but does not affect the sclera, so the nurse should first ask about the child's diet. Carotemia results from increased levels of beta-carotene in the blood, usually related to high dietary intake of yellow-orange foods, such as sweet potatoes and carrots. Carotemia is common in children if caregivers give the child large amounts of carrots but can also occur in adult vegetarians or people who take excessive carotene nutritional supplements.

46. 20 weeks: While the fetal heartbeat may be observed on ultrasound at about 6½ weeks gestation, it cannot usually be detected by fetoscope until 20 weeks. In early pregnancy, fetal heart tones are often more easily heard above the symphysis pubis, but this position shifts later according to fetal growth and position. Fetal heart tones are more easily detected through the fetus's back, so at later weeks of gestation, the nurse should palpate the fetal position before auscultating.

47. 2: In the traditional Hispanic culture, people often believe that children should be started on regular foods early as it will promote increased growth and development, because a common belief is that a large baby is healthier and stronger even though this practice may, in fact, limit growth and increased risk of choking. Some people also believe that the infant must be exposed to cultural foods early to acquire a taste for them. It can be challenging to change cultural ideas, but the nurse should provide as much education about infant nutritional needs as possible.

48. 3: The lower border of the blood pressure cuff should be placed at about 2.5 cm above the antecubital crease. The arm should be flexed slightly at the elbow and positioned so that the antecubital crease is at heart level. The inflatable bladder of the cuff should be over the brachial artery. The nurse should palpate the radial pulse while increasing pressure on the cuff, and when the pulse is no longer palpable, raise cuff pressure another 30 mm Hg.

49. 1: Careful observation can detect hearing deficits at an early age. By 3 months, an infant should exhibit a positive Moro reflex (startle) to sound and may awaken with noise and react to sound by opening or blinking the eyes. Between 3 and 6 months, and infant should begin to coo and try to emulate sounds and should look in the direction of sounds, such as a ringing telephone, and should begin to respond to his or her name. Babies usually begin to say first words by 12 to 15 months, imitate sounds, and follow vocal directions.

50. 1: The symptoms are consistent with diabetes mellitus type 1, so the laboratory assessment that is most indicated is blood glucose and HbA1c. The blood glucose level indicates the current level of glucose in the blood (normal value ≤100 mg/dL), but the level may fluctuate throughout the day and vary according to dietary intake. HbA1c provides a more accurate assessment because it shows the average glucose level over a 3-month period. The normal value for HbA1c is <6%.

51. 1: Hypernatremia results from water deprivation, such as can occur with dehydration, watery diarrhea, burns, diabetes insipidus, heatstroke, and excess sodium chloride administration. Indications include increased serum sodium level (>145 mEq/L) but decreased urine sodium as sodium is reabsorbed by the body rather than excreted through the urine. Urine specific gravity and osmolality are increased because sodium retention results in fluid retention (as the body attempts to compensate) and concentrated urine. Normal value: 135–145 mEq/L; Hyponatremia: <135 mEq/L; Hypernatremia: >145 mEq/L.

52. 2 and 3: Roseola is a contagious disease for which there is no vaccine. It occurs primarily in children between 6 and 24 months of age after the decline of maternal antibodies makes them more susceptible to infection. Roseola is contagious with onset of fever, so the child has been exposed to the virus and may still develop the infection, as the incubation period is 9 to 10 days. Roseola is characterized by high fever for 3 to 8 days followed by a pale pink maculopapular rash that lasts 1 to 2 days.

53. 1: Alginate dressings are appropriate for wounds with a large amount of exudate as they absorb the discharge and form a hydrophilic gel that conforms to the shape of the wound. Because the dressing material (wafers, ropes, fibers) swells in contact with discharge, the wound should be packed loosely. The alginate is covered with a secondary dressing. Hydrocolloid dressings are effective for clean wounds or those with small to moderate exudate. Hydrogel is for dry wounds or those with a small amount of exudate. Transparent film is used with dry wounds.

54. 2 and 3: During a severe generalized tonic-clonic seizure, the client should be turned to side-lying position to prevent aspiration. Padded tongue blades are no longer utilized with seizures and may cause damage to the mouth and teeth. The side rails should be elevated during the seizure and padded, using pillows or blankets, to prevent a fall from the bed and other injuries. The nurse should not physically restrain a client during a seizure as this may cause injury.

55. 4: The Unna boot provides support to the calf muscle pump when the client ambulates, so it cannot be used for clients who are not ambulatory. In this case, it should be discontinued until the client is able to resume ambulation but should be replaced with an alternate form of compression, such as compression stockings, to decrease the danger of deep vein thrombosis. Short stretch wrap, such as Comprilan®, is also used only with ambulatory clients.

56. Metric weight measures

Milligram	Centigram	1-II Decigram	2-I Gram	3-III Dekagram	4-IV Hectogram	Kilogram

57. 2, 3, and 4: This is a sigmoid colostomy, so much of the reabsorptive properties of the colon remain. Because of this, the stool may range from soft to solid. Many clients only expel stool every 2 to 3 days, so the client needs to find what is normal for him. Clients with sigmoid colostomies can often use irrigations to control bowel movements, and some are even able to trigger movements with certain foods or to expel stool on a predictable schedule. Clients should be advised of all of the options for appliances and stoma covers.

58. 3: While over-medication, delirium, and hypoglycemia may all result in weakness and confusion, when the client was asked to show her teeth, the lips clearly lifted more on the left side than on the right side and more teeth can be observed on the left side. This suggests a weakness or paralysis, consistent with a stroke. Since the weakness is on the right side, the stroke is on the left side. When assessing a stroke patient for facial palsy, the nurse can ask the patient to show her teeth or pantomime the action.

59. 2 and 3: With peripheral arterial insufficiency, the foot exhibits rubor on dependency and pallor on elevation. The skin often feels cool and appears pale and shiny with loss of hair on the leg, foot, and toes. Because of impaired circulation, the toenails may appear thick and ridged. Pedal pulses are weak or absent. Ulcers tend to occur on the tips of toes or between toes and on heels or other pressure areas. Ulcers are usually deep, circular, and painful and may be necrotic. Because the venous system may be intact, peripheral edema is usually minimal.

60. 1: Because the onset of symptoms is rapid, these findings are consistent with pulmonary embolism. Acute pulmonary embolism occurs when a thrombus from the venous system or the right side of the heart travels to the lungs and blocks a pulmonary artery or arteriole, resulting in increased alveolar dead space in which ventilation occurs but gas exchange is impaired because of ventilation/perfusion mismatching or intrapulmonary shunting. Common originating sites for thrombus formation are the deep veins in the legs, the pelvic veins, and the right atrium.

61. 3 and 4: The nurse should never attempt to push protruding viscera back through an incision but should examine the viscera for indications of ischemia or other tissue damage and cover it with normal saline–soaked dressings to protect the tissue. The client should be placed in low Fowler's position with head of bed elevated 15 to 45 degrees and knees slightly flexed to reduce tension on the abdominal wound. The client's vital signs must be monitored carefully at least every 15 minutes and the client reassured.

62. 1: The initial intervention when a client reports disturbed sleeping is to complete an assessment of sleep patterns. This should involve questions regarding hours of sleep, quality of sleep, arousals, as well as the number and duration of naps during the day. The client may be asked to keep a sleep diary around the clock, recording sleeping and awakening times, for a few days. Some other initial conservative interventions may include limiting naps and increasing daytime activity, limiting caffeine, maintaining room heat at 70° to 75°F, and playing soft soothing music at bedtime.

63. 2: The client needs to understand the critical importance of using the CPAP machine every time he sleeps. The client's frequent yawning probably indicates that he is not using the machine routinely. Obstructive sleep apnea is characterized by passive collapse of the pharynx during sleep because of upper airway narrowing, often associated with obesity. Patients usually snore loudly with cycles of breath cessation caused by apneic periods lasting up to 60 seconds. These may occur 30 or more times a night despite continued chest wall and abdominal movements, indicating an automatic attempt to breathe.

64. 1 and 3: With continuous ambulatory peritoneal dialysis (CAPD) the client instills about 2 liters of fluid over 10 to 15 minutes and then clamps the tubing and folds the tubing and bag over the abdomen and secures it with clothing, maintaining a dwell time of 3 to 5 hours. After this, the tubing is unclamped and dialysate and waste products drained for about 20 minutes. This drainage is discarded and new dialysate instilled to begin the cycle again.

65. 1: The blood abnormalities of most concern during treatment of leukemia and most other cancers as well are thrombocytopenia and neutropenia. About 10% of clients with ALL initially present with disseminated intravascular coagulation (DIC) because of thrombocytopenia. As the platelet level falls, the ability of the blood to clot is impaired and the client is at risk for hemorrhage. The absolute neutrophil count is monitored closely because, as the ANC falls, the risk for exogenous and endogenous infections increases markedly.

66. 1: Hypoparathyroidism with hypocalcemia is a complication of thyroidectomy. Hypocalcemia may occur because of inadvertent removal of all or some of the parathyroid glands but may also occur temporarily after surgery because of edema or manipulation of the parathyroid glands during the thyroidectomy. Typical symptoms include a tingling sensation about the mouth and in the fingers and toes. Some may develop severe muscle cramps and tetany. Transient mild

31

hypoparathyroidism may require no treatment, but IV calcium gluconate is indicated for calcium levels below 7 mg/dL.

67. 4: The meal that most corresponds to the dietary guidelines is one-half banana, 1 cup broccoli, ½ cup quinoa, 3 ounces roasted turkey, and 8 ounces of 1% milk. The dietary guidelines advise that half of a plate should be filled with fruits and vegetables and that grains should be whole grains (such as quinoa and brown rice). Milk products should be low- or nonfat, and protein should be lean and include limited red meat as well as nonmeat sources of protein, such as beans, eggs, and soy products.

68. 1 and 3: The pre-adolescent child needs to be aware of bodily changes to expect as he develops secondary sexual characteristics, including normal variations among children and changes in height, weight, and body structure. The mother should allow the child to express changes in the way he thinks and awareness and should stress the importance of education. She should also ask the child about issues related to peer pressure, such as bullying, gangs, drugs, tobacco, and alcohol use.

69. 1-IV, 2-I, 3-II, 4-III: The nurse should prepare the child for the treatment by removing all clothes except the diaper so that as much skin as possible is exposed to the light. The nurse should apply a protective mask over the child's eyes and adjust the light source to 15 to 20 cm above the child prior to turning on the lights and administering the treatment. Indications include:

Weight	Serum bilirubin level
500 to 750 g	5 to 8 mg/dL
751 to 1000 g	6 to 10 mg/dL
1001 to 1250 g	8 to 10 mg/dL
1251 to 1500 g	10 to 12 mg/dL

70. 4: A client with a severe cough and fever requires both standard precautions and droplet precautions. The best action is to provide the client with a facemask and seat the client in a separate area as far away from other clients as possible to reduce the chance of the infection spreading. A client who is ill should not be sent away or asked to wait outside. The nurse should thoroughly wash his/her hands after contact with the client.

71. 3: While bedrest alone with much time in the lateral decubitus position to maximize uterine blood flow is often indicated for clients with mild pre-eclampsia, those with severe pre-eclampsia (BP >160–180/>110 and proteinuria >5 g/24 hours) are usually treated initially with magnesium sulfate (IM or IV) as a prophylaxis to prevent seizures. An antihypertensive, such as hydralazine, is given if the diastolic pressure remains above 110. If seizures (eclampsia) occur, magnesium sulfate or other anticonvulsants, such as diazepam and phenytoin, may be used to prevent recurrence.

72. 1: Women who experience premature rupture of the membranes at term and do not go into labor within 12 to 24 hours are induced because the risk of infection increases with time. About 9 out of 10 women with premature rupture of the membranes go into labor within 24 hours. In some cases, such as a woman with a history of current or recent vaginal infection or multiple digital vaginal exams, labor may be induced at any time after the membranes rupture.

73. 1: Pulmonary hygiene is especially important after surgery because inactivity and failure to breathe deeply and cough, aggravated by pain, can result in atelectasis. Patients should be instructed in the use of the incentive spirometer both before surgery and after surgery and use should be monitored to ensure compliance. Patients with atelectasis typically initially become short of breath and may develop a cough and low-grade fever as secretions pool and the lung collapses. Untreated, the patient may develop hypoxemia, pneumonia, or respiratory failure.

74. 4: These symptoms are consistent with mild pacemaker syndrome and occur when the atrial and ventricular contractions are not synchronized properly. This causes decreased cardiac output because the atria do not adequately fill the ventricles. Peripheral vascular resistance increases to compensate initially. Moderate pacemaker syndrome is characterized by increasing dyspnea and orthopnea, dizziness, vertigo, confusion, and sensation of choking. Severe pacemaker syndrome includes pulmonary edema with rales and marked dyspnea, syncope, and heart failure.

75. 4: Clients are often quite nervous about cardiac monitoring, especially if they are fearful about their condition, and they may dislodge leads so that they can get attention from nurses because they are afraid to be alone or need reassurance. Challenging a client or attempting to make the person feel guilty does not solve the underlying problem. A better approach is for the nurse to take time to talk with the client, explaining how telemetry works, what the numbers and tracings on the monitor mean, and what the staff is learning from the monitoring.

76. 1: The nurse should always remember the five rights of delegation: right task, right circumstances, right person, right direction or communication, and right supervision. The nurse should never delegate tasks for which assistive personnel have not been trained, and this includes administration of medications and blood therapy. Assistive personnel can monitor vital signs during blood therapy and should be taught to recognize and report signs of adverse effects, but the responsibility for primary monitoring lies with the nurse.

77. 4: Gastric fluid is acidic, usually with a pH value of 4 or less. Intestinal aspirate is usually greater than 4 and respiratory secretions greater than 5.5. However, the nurse should not rely on pH alone, but should carefully observe the color and consistency of aspirate. Gastric fluids may vary in color from green and cloudy (most common) to white, tan, red-tinged (from blood), or brown. If the tube is placed in the duodenum, aspirate may be yellow or bile-stained. If the end of the NG tube is in the esophagus, the aspirate may be clear and look like saliva.

78. 2: Because the client has systemic symptoms (fever, chills) and flank pain, these symptoms suggest a kidney infection rather than cystitis. The initial diagnostic tests include a urinalysis and urine culture and sensitivities to determine the causative organism. Clients are usually started on a broad-spectrum antibiotic while awaiting the culture and sensitivity report. In most cases, symptoms recede rapidly once antibiotics are started, so if the infection is severe or the client's condition deteriorates, the client may need hospitalization for intravenous antibiotic therapy.

79. 1, 2, and 4: Radiotherapy to the abdominal area and pelvis often damages cells in the intestines, resulting in diarrhea. Clients should be advised to drink 8 to 12 glasses of clear liquids, eat 5 to 6 small meals daily, and limit fiber, fat, and lactose (milk products) as they may increase diarrhea. Some people benefit from the BRAT diet, especially when diarrhea is acute—banana, rice, applesauce, and toast. Clients should also avoid fried and spicy foods, cruciferous vegetables and beans, and soy products.

80. 0.7: The formula for calculating the waist-to-hip ratio is: waist (inches) divided by hips (inches).

In this case 28/40 = 0.7. The waist must be measured at its smallest circumference and the hips at the widest. This measurement determines whether a person's body type is classified as "pear" or "apple." People with "apple" shapes have increased abdominal fat, which is a higher health risk than fat in the hips.

Gender	Ideal	Increased risk	High risk
Male	0.9 to 0.95	0.96 to 1.0	>1.0
Female	0.7 to 0.8	0.81 to 0.85	>0.85

81. 4: If the nurse is planning to empty a Jackson-Pratt drainage device but notes a number of large clots in the tubing, the nurse should milk the tubing to move the clots into the device before emptying it. The nurse may use an alcohol swab to facilitate the process. The nurse begins by pinching off the tubing at the distal end and, using an alcohol swab wrapped around the tubing, squeezing the tubing with fingers of the other hand, and sliding a short distance down the tubing, forcing the clots to move down. This procedure is repeated the length of the tubing.

82. 1, 3, and 4: If the nurse is discussing the use of a condom, information that is important to share includes:

- Use a condom every time for every sexual encounter.
- Use latex rather than natural membrane condoms for better protection.
- Use only water-based lubricants.
- Use spermicide if trying to prevent pregnancy.
- Hold the condom in place when withdrawing the penis after ejaculation.
- Leave a 1-inch space at the end of the condom to contain ejaculate.

The nurse should also demonstrate how the condom is applied, using a model if one is available.

83. 1, 3 and 5: If a client has suffered second-degree burns from falling asleep in the sun and states she sunbathes 8 to 10 hours a week to maintain a tan, the advice that is most important to share is that excessive exposure to the sun increases the risk of skin cancer, and self-tanners are available that do not require sun exposure. Current guidelines suggest that exposing the bare skin for 20 minutes daily is safe and adequate for production of vitamin D. The client should apply sunscreen for exposure of longer duration.

84. 150 minutes: Current exercise guidelines for adults recommend that they engage in strengthening exercises, such as weight training, twice weekly. They should also engage in aerobic activities of at least 150 minutes per week for moderate activities, such as swimming and walking, or 75 minutes per week of vigorous activities (such as running or aerobic dancing). Clients may be encouraged to join an exercise group or a local gym to encourage compliance.

85. The correct order for the clean intermittent catheterization (CIC) procedure is as follows:

1: (Step 1) III. Spread labia and cleanse area with soap and water.
2: (Step 2) I. Locate meatus (by touch or by using a mirror).
3: (Step 3) IV. Lubricate catheter (with water-soluble lubricant)
4: (Step 4) II. Insert catheter and hold in place until urine stops draining.

The catheter is then removed and discarded if disposable or cleaned according to manufacturer's directions for future use.

86. 3: If the nurse is a member of a team in which two members have an escalating personal conflict that is affecting team morale and functioning, the initial response should be to express concern to the two (discussing how it is affecting the team) and offer to mediate. The nurse should listen to both sides of the issue and try to help them reach a resolution. If the nurses refuse or the conflict continues, then the nurse should report the situation to the unit supervisor.

87. 1: The Wong-Baker FACES pain scale is likely the most effective pain scale for assessing pain in a 6-year-old child. FACES can be used for children from about 4 to 16 and also for some adults, especially older adults. FACES comes in both a pediatric and an adult version. Children with normal cognitive ability can usually understand the numeric pain intensity scale by about age 8. The CRIES scale is used for infants and the PAINAD scale for clients with dementia.

88. 4: While all of these statements may lead to a discussion about feelings and better management of pain, the statement that suggests a need for education is: "I know all this morphine is making her a drug addict." At one time, healthcare providers withheld pain medication from cancer patients in the mistaken belief that they would become addicts, but the spouse needs to understand the difference between taking narcotics for pleasure and for palliation.

89. 3: The WBC and platelet counts are outside normal range:

Test	Result	Normal value
WBC	4.1	4.8-10.8 (10^3/µL)
RBC	4.38	4.20-5.40 (10^6/µL)
Hemoglobin	13.8	12.0-16.0 (g/dL)
Hematocrit	42.0	37.0-47.0 (%)
Platelet count	116	150-450 (10^3/µL)

90. 1: If a client has had a stroke in the right hemisphere and has weakness on the left side, expressive aphasia, and some dysphagia, the most appropriate referral is to a speech and language therapist because these professionals are trained to assess dysphagia and provide therapy to improve the ability to swallow. The speech and language therapist may use a number of different strategies to improve swallowing (sensory, thermal, suck-swallow, strengthening exercises), and can provide guidance to staff on compensatory methods to reduce risk of aspiration.

91. 4: If, when inserting a nasogastric feeding tube, the nurse pauses after inserting the tube 25 cm, this is at the level of the carina. If the nurse listens at the distal end of the tube and hears air exchange, this is an indication that the tube is in the respiratory tract and not the esophagus. The tube should be immediately completely withdrawn, allowing the client time to relax and stop coughing, before insertion is attempted again. Note, even if there is no sound of air exchange, this cannot be used as confirmation of correct placement.

92. 1, 2, 4, and 5: Signs and symptoms consistent with diabetes mellitus, type 1, include the following:

- 3 Ps—polyuria, polydipsia, and polyphagia as the body tries to compensate for the increased glucose level.
- Recent weight loss: This occurs because protein and stored fat is broken down because of the body's inability to utilize glucose for energy.
- Weakness, fatigue: Inadequate glucose stores to provide energy needs.
- Blurred vision: Caused by increased fluid in the lens of the eye.
- Kussmaul breathing: Hyperventilation that occurs with diabetic ketoacidosis.

93. If the nurse must sit a patient who is lying supine in a hospital bed onto the side of the bed in preparation for transfer to a wheelchair, the steps to this procedure are:

1: (First): III. Raise head of bed to 30°.
2: (Second) I. Roll client onto side, facing nurse.
3: (Third) II. Place one hand under shoulders and the other over the hips.
4: (Fourth) Pivot the client into a sitting position.

The nurse must be sure to maintain proper alignment of the client's body and to use correct body mechanics to avoid injuries.

94. 2: If a client who is receiving total parenteral nutrition (TPN) has weakness and dizziness and is diaphoretic, pale, lethargic, and increasingly confused, the laboratory test that is most indicated is serum glucose because these signs and symptoms are consistent with hypoglycemia. Hypoglycemia is a common complication of TPN and may result from too much insulin. Insulin should be stopped and dextrose concentration increased as well as rate of infusion slowed until the client stabilizes. The client should also be evaluated for sepsis because hypoglycemia may be a symptom.

95. 1: The most therapeutic response to a client in the cardiac care unit who is upset since two other clients in the unit died and tells the nurse, "Everyone dies here. I don't know why you are bothering treating me," is to respond with: "You are worried that you are going to die." This is stating in concrete terms what the client is implying and giving the client the opportunity to discuss the concerns.

96. 3: If a nurse is floated to the oncology unit but has not had previous experience administering IV chemotherapy, which the nurse must administer to two clients, the most appropriate response is to discuss the lack of experience with the unit supervisor, who should adjust the assignment or assign another nurse to assist. The nurse should express a willingness to learn, but should be honest about limitations; failing to do so may result in injury to a client.

97. 1: Because this type of injury is almost always the result on abuse and not an accident, the nurse should report the incident to Child Protective Services according to state guidelines, as nurses are mandatory reporters of child abuse. The nurse should not attempt to question the child, who is already traumatized, or confront the parents, as this could result in their immediately attempting to remove the child from the emergency department or reacting violently.

98. 1: If the nurse observed another nurse remove a hydrocodone tablet from a client's medicine drawer and then swallow the tablet when it appeared no one was looking, the most appropriate response is to immediately report the incident to a direct supervisor. The nurse should not attempt to confront the nurse or counsel the nurse, as the nurse who took the drug is likely to deny doing so and may become agitated and angry.

99. 2: If a 38-year-old client with rheumatoid arthritis is having increasing difficulty dressing herself and managing activities of daily living at home because of her disabilities, the referral that may be most effective is an occupational therapist. Occupational therapists can assess the client's needs and assist the client to improve fine motor skills or compensate for the loss of those skills. The occupational therapist can provide guidance regarding assistive devices and performance of activities of daily living.

100. 1, 3, and 4: Motivational interviewing is a nonconfrontational communication approach. Important elements of motivational interviewing include:

- Express empathy instead of criticism.
- Focus on client's strengths, not weaknesses.
- Avoid confrontation.
- Listen instead of giving advice.
- Recognize that change is the client's responsibility.
- Adjust to resistance from the client rather than oppose.
- Help client recognize gap between current situation and goals.

101. 1, 2, and 3: If a client is exhibiting local manifestations of inflammation about a wound, the following characteristics of inflammation are evident:

- Pain/Tenderness: changes in pH, nerve stimulation, and pressure from exudate result in increased pain
- Edema: fluid shifts to interstitial spaces and accumulates in the tissue
- Rubor: vasodilation causes the tissue to appear pink/red tinged
- Heat: increased metabolism results in increase of temperature in the inflamed tissue; release of cytokines may cause body temperature to rise

102. 1: Because this is the first time that the parents will place the infant in a car seat, the nurse should check the installation to make sure that the car seat is properly secured. Then, the nurse should question the parents to ensure that they know how to position the infant in the car seat, providing education and helpful advice as necessary, and finally should observe as the parents position the newborn in the car seat.

103. 1 and 4: If a client tells the nurse that his physician has advised him to take OTC anti-inflammatory drugs to control the discomfort of osteoarthritis but the client is unsure what that means, the nurse should advise the client that NSAIDs, such as ibuprofen, and salicylates, such as aspirin, are OTC anti-inflammatory drugs. Acetaminophen is an antipyretic rather than an anti-inflammatory drug and may help to reduce both pain and fever. Corticosteroids require prescriptions.

104. 3: If a client has a large pressure sore and is suffering from malnutrition and has had little protein in her diet, this slows the healing process because of the lack of amino acids needed to repair tissue. Clients with wounds need extra protein to promote the healing process, so the client should be carefully assessed by a nutritionist to determine an adequate diet. Usual requirements for healing are 1.25 to 1.5 g/kg/day of protein.

105. 2: The client's pressure sore is stage II. Wound staging:

- Stage I: localized intact skin with nonblanchable redness
- Stage II: partial thickness loss of dermis and red/pink wound surface without slough
- Stage III: full thickness loss of dermis with subcutaneous tissue exposed. Slough, undermining and tunneling may be present.
- Stage IV: full thickness loss of dermis with muscle, tendons, or bones exposed. Slough or eschar may be present.

106. When examining a client's abdomen, the nurse would expect to find the following abdominal structures in the quadrants below:

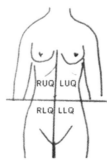

- RUQ: III. Liver and gallbladder
- LUQ: I. Spleen
- RLQ: IV. Cecum and appendix
- LLQ: II. Sigmoid flexure (descending colon)

107. 124 grams: If a client who is receiving total parenteral nutrition (TPN) must receive 2 grams of protein per kilogram of body weight each day and the patient's weight is 136.4 lb, the first step is to convert pounds into kilograms: 136.4/2.2 = 62. Then the total number of kilograms is multiplied by the required grams per kilogram to find the daily total: 62 × 2 = 124 grams. Most clients receive 1.5 to 2 g/kg/day in TPN solutions.

108. 4: If a client reports being allergic to kiwi fruit, bananas, and avocados, the client is especially at risk for allergy to latex, so latex products should be avoided. The proteins in these foods are similar to those in latex, resulting in the latex-food syndrome. Clients with a history of exposure to latex at work or in health care are also at increased risk. Allergic reactions can range from mild to severe, and can include rash, urticaria, erythema, asthma-like symptoms, and anaphylaxis.

109. 1, 2, 3, and 4: Guillain-Barré syndrome, diabetes mellitus type 1, rheumatoid arthritis, and Hashimoto thyroiditis are all examples of autoimmune disorders. An autoimmune disorder is one in which the client's immune system attacks body tissue. The immune disorder may be systemic, such as with rheumatoid arthritis, or more localized, such as with Hashimoto thyroiditis. About 80 diseases have been identified as autoimmune disorders. Autoimmune disorders often have periods of remission in which symptoms subside, followed by exacerbation of symptoms.

110. 3: If a nurse notes that a portable electrocardiogram machine (or any machine) has a frayed electrical cord, the nurse must immediately remove the machine from service, following established protocols. Because of the danger of fire, placing a sign (which may be ignored) on the machine, or leaving the machine and making a report to the unit supervisor are not adequate. The nurse should never place any tape—even electrical tape—around a frayed cord. The cord must be replaced.

111. Triage order:

- (First) II. 16-year-old male with chest injury in respiratory distress and severe pain. (Because ABCs are attended to first.)
- (Second) IV. Very agitated, hallucinating, and confused middle-aged male with unknown injuries reeking of alcohol. (Because the client poses risk to self and others and may have head injury or severe undetected injury.)

- (Third) I. 64-year old woman, alert and responsive, with large laceration of the head. (Because of possible undetected underlying head injury.)
- (Fourth) III. 28-year-old male with multiple contusions and fractured right arm. (Last because these injuries are not likely life-threatening.)

112. 4: If a client with osteomyelitis of the right tibia that has cultured positive for *Staphylococcus aureus* is to be discharged home with dressing changes done daily by nurses from a home health agency, the most important point to stress about infection control is handwashing. The client and family members should be instructed in proper handwashing technique and the use of alcohol-based hand scrubs. Since a dressing is in place, gowns and gloves are not necessary for all contact with the client. The environmental surfaces should be kept clean.

113. 1: If a nurse must move a heavy cart full of supplies, the technique that uses the best body mechanics is to push the cart from behind with both hands, keeping the head up, back straight, and knees bent to prevent muscle injury. The nurse should avoid pulling or twisting when moving items and should stand close to the item that is being pushed rather than standing at a distance and leaning into it.

114. 2: Generally, the faster the gait, the greater the ambulation speed, the greater expenditure of energy and need for strength. If this 19-year-old client wants to keep pace with his friends and is sufficiently strong and stable, then the fastest gait is the swing-through gate. Procedure: Bear weight on good foot, move both crutches forward, swing both legs through and past the crutches, landing on the good foot. The slowest gait (and the one that requires the least energy) is the 4-point alternate gate.

115. 4: The best method to properly adjust a walker to the correct height for a client is to have the client stand with arms dangling at the side and then to measure the distance from the client's wrists to the floor. This is the height to which the walker (at the handles) should be adjusted. Walkers are intended for partial weight-bearing only and are not meant to support a client's full weight.

116. 3:

This symbol represents biohazards and is affixed to sharps containers because needles and other sharps may be contaminated with blood or other body fluids. Materials that are labeled with the biohazard symbol must be handled properly and disposed of in such a way as to render the biological material inert and noninfectious. Waste that is a biohazard must be contained in puncture-resistant bags or containers. Different disposal methods for biohazardous materials include incineration, steam sterilization, and chemical disinfection.

117. 2: Even though a medication error may seem relatively harmless, any time an error is made, the proper procedures must be followed. These include notifying the client's physician, documenting the actual medication given on the client's record (without indicating that it was given in error), and filing an incident report that describes in detail how the incident occurred. Individual institutions may have specific reporting protocols that must be followed, such as requiring a report to risk management or a supervisor.

118. 1: If a client who had abdominal surgery the previous day experiences evisceration and the nurse finds intestines protruding from the wound, the initial step that the nurse should take to protect the wound is to cover it with saline-soaked sterile dressings to keep the tissue moist and prevent irritation. Evisceration requires emergent surgical intervention to prevent sepsis. The head of the bed should be elevated to semi-Fowler's position and the knees slightly flexed to reduce tension on the wound.

119. 3: If the nurse is working in a hospital unit when a tornado creates mass casualties and the hospital is on alert and advising staff that hospital beds must be freed for incoming injured, the nurse should immediately begin to make a list of noncritical clients who might be safely discharged so that discharge plans can be made quickly if the need arises. The nurse should avoid calling physicians and tying up the phone lines until receiving more specific information.

120. 4: Because naloxone (Narcan) reverses the action of opioids, if administered to a long-time opioid user, it may trigger a severe withdrawal reaction and seizures. The dosage of naloxone should be titrated carefully and the client monitored throughout treatment. Withdrawal symptoms may occur within minutes of administration of the drug, depending on the dosage of medication and the degree of opioid dependence.

Practice Test #2

1. A client with Alzheimer's disease is hospitalized after a mild stroke. The client calls out frequently and often tries to climb out of bed. What is the best room assignment for the client?

    1. a private room within the line of sight of the nursing station
    2. a private room at the end of the hallway away from other, more critically ill, clients
    3. a shared room with another cognitively impaired client
    4. any room as long as the client is physically restrained

2. Which of the following is the most effective method for reducing the spread of nosocomial infections, such as *Clostridium difficile?*

    1. placing clients in private rooms
    2. providing antibiotic prophylaxis
    3. cleaning the rooms with a disinfectant
    4. practicing a thorough, consistent handwashing routine

3. A client with chronic lower back pain asks the nurse if she might benefit from some type of complementary therapy. Which of the following complementary therapies should the nurse discuss with the client? Select all that apply.

    1. massage
    2. aromatherapy
    3. homeopathy
    4. acupuncture
    5. visualization and relaxation

4. Following the death of a client, the nurse anticipates that rigor mortis will begin in what period of time?

    1. four to six hours
    2. two to four hours
    3. one to two hours
    4. 30 to 60 minutes

5. Regarding examination of the abdomen, which anatomic structures are found in the different abdominal quadrants?

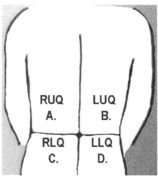

RUQ A. | LUQ B.
RLQ C. | LLQ D.

I. Cecum and appendix.
II. Spleen.
III. Liver and gallbladder.
IV. Sigmoid colon.

Place the structures (in Roman numerals) into the correct quadrants.

1. (RUQ)
2. (LUQ)
3. (RLQ)
4. (LLQ)

6. Epinephrine is supplied for a nebulizer inhaler in a dosage of 1:100. What is the percentage strength of the solution? *Record your answer using a whole number.*

7. When administering total parenteral nutrition (TPN) to a client, how often should the nurse change the filters, intravenous (IV) tubing, and solution?

a. every 8 hours
b. every 12 hours
c. every 24 hours
d. every 48 hours

8. The Tensilon® (edrophonium chloride) test is used to diagnose which of the following?

1. myasthenia gravis
2. multiple sclerosis
3. Parkinson's disease
4. Bell's palsy

9. A client is to have continuous measuring of oxygen saturation with a pulse oximeter, but he has a constant tremor of both of his hands and he tends to pick at the covers. Which of the following is the best solution?

1. apply the oximeter to the little finger because the tremors will not interfere
2. apply the oximeter to the little finger, and tape it in place
3. advise the physician that pulse oximetry is not possible
4. apply an earlobe oximeter

10. A client with extensive burns of the lower extremities is treated with topical agents, and the burns are wrapped with several layers of dressings. On examination, the nurse finds that the peripheral pulses are diminished. Which is the best initial action for the nurse?

1. elevate the extremities to reduce edema
2. remove the dressings
3. loosen the dressings
4. reevaluate the peripheral pulses after 15 minutes

11. A client with uterine cancer is receiving intracavity irradiation with an intrauterine "stem" device. On examination, the nurse discovers that the radiation source has become dislodged and is partially outside of the vagina. Which action should the nurse carry out?

1. wear rubber gloves to lift the stem and place it in a shielded container
2. immediately notify the radiation department
3. cover the stem with a folded towel to protect the client's skin
4. use rubber gloves to gently reinsert the stem into the vagina

12. A 58-year-old client is to be discharged after hip replacement surgery. What adaptive equipment does the nurse expect that the client will need initially in the home? Select all that apply.

1. walker
2. elevated toilet seat
3. wheelchair
4. reacher/grabber
5. sock aid

13. A train accident has resulted in many severe casualties, and the emergency department is inundated with clients, but few hospital beds are available. What is the best solution to this emergency situation?

1. transfer incoming clients to other facilities as soon as they are stabilized
2. place newly admitted clients in the hallways
3. close the emergency room to further clients
4. carry out early discharge for low-risk, noncritical clients to free up some beds

14. A client has end-stage renal disease (ESRD). Which of the following diagnostic findings are consistent with ESRD? Select all that apply.

1. decreased creatinine clearance
2. metabolic acidosis
3. respiratory acidosis
4. anemia
5. hypophosphatemia
6. hypercalcemia

15. A client receiving chemotherapy for ovarian cancer works for a small company with six employees and asks the nurse if she is allowed accommodations at work because of her cancer under provisions of the Americans with Disabilities Act (ADA). Which is the best response?

    1. "The company must accommodate your needs under provisions of the ADA."
    2. "The company is exempt from the provisions of the ADA because of its size."
    3. "The company must allow you time for treatment but can require you to continue to work full time."
    4. "Cancer is not considered a disability, so the provisions of the ADA do not apply."

16. When conducting a physical exam and assessing the apical pulse in an adult client, where should the nurse place the stethoscope?

    1. second left intercostal space at the midclavicular line
    2. fourth left intercostal space at the sternal margin
    3. fourth left intercostal space at the midclavicular line
    4. fifth left intercostal space at the midclavicular line

17. A client with breast cancer who has the BRCA1 gene, which is transmitted in an autosomal-dominant manner, asks the nurse if her children are likely to inherit the gene. Which of the following information should the nurse provide?

    1. each child has a 25% chance of inheriting the gene
    2. each child has a 50% chance of inheriting the gene
    3. all children will inherit the gene
    4. no children will inherit the gene

18. A client who has been taking oral prednisone to control his chronic obstructive pulmonary disease (COPD) wants to transition to inhaled corticosteroids. The nurse anticipates which of the following scenarios?

    1. the client must be tapered from the oral drug while beginning treatment with the inhaled drug
    2. the client must be tapered from the oral drug before beginning treatment with the inhaled drug
    3. the oral medication can be discontinued immediately, and the client can be started on the inhaled drug
    4. the oral medication cannot be discontinued, so the client cannot transition to the inhaled drug

19. A client has been diagnosed with Parkinson's disease. Which of the following findings would the nurse expect to observe? Select all that apply.

    1. resting tremor (unilateral)
    2. flaccidity
    3. hyperkinesia
    4. postural instability
    5. dysphagia
    6. flat affect

20. A child weighing 30 kg is being treated with Zosyn® (piperacillin/tazobactam) IV every eight hours with a dose of 100 mg piperacillin/12.5 mg tazobactam per kg of body weight. What is the child's correct dosage in grams (g)?

  1. 3000 g piperacillin/375 g tazobactam
  2. 30 g piperacillin/37.5 g tazobactam
  3. 3 g piperacillin/3.75 g tazobactam
  4. 3 g piperacillin/0.375 g tazobactam

21. A client has been admitted to the mental health unit for bipolar disorder. On the care plan, the nurse has listed "chronic low self-esteem" as a nursing diagnosis with "self-esteem enhancement" and "self-awareness enhancement" as interventions. Which of the following would the nurse include as expected outcomes? Select all that apply.

  1. the client is able to use positive self-talk to interrupt negative thinking
  2. the client is able to develop strategies to increase his interactions with others
  3. the client is able to verbalize the symptoms of bipolar disorder and the treatments
  4. the client is able to use positive coping behaviors to improve his functioning
  5. the client is able to develop satisfying personal relationships

22. A nine-year-old boy weighing 22 kg is to receive 15 mg of gabapentin per kilogram of body weight daily in three divided doses to control seizures. How many milligrams will he receive in each dose? *Record your answer using a whole number.*

23. A client receiving oral tetracycline for the treatment of acne should be advised to avoid which of the following?

  1. sunbathing
  2. swimming
  3. running
  4. weight lifting

24. The nurse is instructing a client with Addison's disease (adrenocortical insufficiency) about the signs and symptoms of Addisonian crisis. Which of the following should the nurse include? Select all that apply.

  1. hypertension
  2. pallor
  3. bradycardia
  4. nausea and abdominal pain
  5. tachycardia
  6. confusion and restlessness

25. A client receiving chemotherapy for breast cancer is to receive metoclopramide HCl at the dosage of 2 mg/kg of body weight 30 minutes before chemotherapy. If the client weighs 55 kg and the medication is provided with 5 mg per milliliter, how many milliliters of medication should the client receive? Record your answer using a whole number.

26. A 48-year-old female client complains of episodes of severe right upper quadrant abdominal pain lasting two to six hours, indigestion, nausea and vomiting, and clay-colored stools. The nurse suspects the client may have which of the following diagnoses?

1. colitis
2. pancreatitis
3. cholecystitis
4. diverticulitis

27. When the nurse is doing a physical exam, which part of his hand is most sensitive to temperature variations?

1. thumb
2. fingertips
3. palm
4. dorsum

28. A 90-year-old client with moderate Alzheimer's disease lives with her son and daughter-in-law. Which statement by the daughter-in-law suggests a need for more education about the disease?

1. "She purposely hides her belongings from me."
2. "I have to keep the doors latched at all times."
3. "She thinks I'm her mother at times."
4. "She can't remember where the bathroom is located."

29. The nurse has used a needle and syringe to add medication to an intravenous (IV) solution. Which of the following actions should the nurse carry out after injecting the medication into the solution?

1. invert the IV bag briefly
2. begin the infusion with no further action
3. roll the IV bag back and forth between the hands a few times
4. gently shake the IV bag

30. The client is to use a metered-dose inhaler (MDI) without a spacer for albuterol. How should the nurse advise the client to position the inhaler for self-administration?

1. in her mouth with her lips sealed around the opening
2. touching her lips but outside of the mouth
3. one to two inches in front of her mouth
4. three to four inches in front of her mouth

31. A client with pancreatic cancer is prescribed fentanyl patches to control pain. Which statement by the client indicates the need for more education?

1. "The patch will give better pain control if I apply heat over it."
2. "I should rotate the sites of administration."
3. "I can dispose of the patch by rolling it up and flushing it down the toilet."
4. "I should cover the patch with plastic when showering."

32. Which of the following drugs is the appropriate antidote for an overdose of acetaminophen?

1. protamine sulfate
2. folic acid
3. naloxone
4. *N*-acetylcysteine

33. A client has been prescribed 96 mg of theophylline, which is available as 80 mg per 15 mL. How many milliliters should the client receive? *Record your answer using a whole number.*

34. The nurse notes that a client has slid down onto the floor, and he is unable to get up. Which of the following is the best method of lifting him?

1. belt lift
2. mechanical lift
3. two-person chicken lift (lifting under the client's arms)
4. blanket lift

35. The nurse believes that the dosage of a medication is too high for a client, based on the recommended milligrams per kilogram of weight. Which of the following initial actions should the nurse carry out?

1. contact the pharmacy to determine if the dosage is within acceptable limits
2. notify the supervisor of her concerns
3. telephone the physician to question the dosage
4. assume the dosage was verified when ordered, and administer the drug

36. Which of the following descriptions fit the profile of an infant abductor? Select all that apply.

1. female, approximately age 30
2. male, approximately age 30
3. a frequent visitor to the nursery
4. a visitor who asks many questions about nursery and hospital procedures
5. a frequent, friendly visitor who chats with staff and parents, getting to know them
6. a person with a criminal record

37. The nurse agrees to represent the hospital at a job fair, distributing alcohol-based hand cleansers to participants and telling them about methods of preventing the flu. Which of the following does this participation primarily represent?

1. professional development
2. community health education
3. community service
4. hospital promotion

38. An eight-year-old client lives with his married parents, siblings, grandparents, two aunts, and a cousin. Which of the following family types does this situation comprise?

1. nuclear family
2. coparenting
3. extended family
4. extended kin network

39. The nurse is to administer 250 mL of normal saline intravenously with a flow rate of 15 drops per minute and a drop factor of 15 drops/mL. How many minutes will it take to complete the infusion? *Record your answer using a whole number.*

40. The physician has ordered wrist restraints for a client who is confused and combative and attempting to pull out her Foley catheter. Which of the following actions can the nurse delegate to unlicensed assistive personnel? Select all that apply.
    1. application of restraints
    2. assessing the continued need for restraints
    3. reviewing the correct placement of restraints
    4. repositioning the client while in restraints
    5. decision regarding the type of restraints needed

41. The nurse is completing the health history with a client, and he appears obviously uncomfortable when the nurse asks questions about sexuality. Which of the following is the best method of dealing with the client's discomfort?
    1. acknowledge the client's discomfort in a supportive manner
    2. make a casual joke, stating that everyone feels discomfort talking about personal issues
    3. stop asking about sexuality and continue with the next part of the history
    4. ignore the client's discomfort

42. When the nurse enters the break room, she finds that a colleague is sharing personal information about his client with other staff members. What is the best action for the nurse?
    1. leave the break room
    2. report the situation to a supervisor
    3. tell the colleague that he should not be talking about a client
    4. tell the colleague and staff members that you are not comfortable violating a client's privacy

43. A client has had a Port-a-Cath inserted in the upper chest and is receiving chemotherapy, but the client is very tense and complains of much discomfort when the port is accessed. Which of the following is the best solution to the client's discomfort?
    1. administer pain medication prior to the treatment
    2. apply EMLA cream prior to the treatment
    3. inject a local anesthetic prior to the treatment
    4. instruct the client in deep-breathing and relaxation techniques

44. The nurse is to do chest physiotherapy on an eight-year-old child with cystic fibrosis. Which lobes of the lung are being treated if the child is lying prone with a pillow under the abdomen and lower legs and percussion is administered at the base of the scapulae and immediately inferior to the scapulae?
    1. posterior segments of the right and left upper lobes
    2. anterior segments of the right and left lower lobes
    3. superior segments of the right and left lower lobes
    4. apical segments of the right and left upper lobes

45. The nurse is caring for a client who is undergoing peritoneal dialysis. How long does the nurse expect that a typical exchange cycle (infusion, dwell time, and drainage) will take to complete?

    1. 12 hours
    2. 3 to 4 hours
    3. 60 to 90 minutes
    4. 30 to 45 minutes

46. A pregnant woman admitted for preeclampsia experiences a seizure. In what position should the nurse place the client during the seizure?

    1. supine semi-Fowler's position
    2. right lateral
    3. supine flat position
    4. left lateral

47. A client receiving radiation to the abdomen complains of almost-constant diarrhea. Which of the following should the client do to manage diarrhea? Select all that apply.

    1. drink eight or more cups of clear liquids daily
    2. increase intake of high-fiber foods
    3. drink three to four cups of milk daily
    4. eat five to six small meals daily
    5. take Imodium® as prescribed
    6. use baby wipes to cleanse the rectal area

48. Under which delivery care model would the nurse expect to be responsible for the least number of clients?

    1. functional
    2. total patient care
    3. team nursing
    4. modified primary care

49. What is the nurse's primary responsibility related to continuous quality performance improvement?

    1. the nurse should cooperate with measures designed to improve performance
    2. the nurse should be informed about methods of continuous quality performance improvement
    3. the nurse should actively seek methods to improve performance
    4. the nurse should help evaluate outcomes of quality performance improvement measures

50. A client with a new hearing aid complains of acoustic feedback—whistling—that prevents him from hearing. What should the nurse advise as the initial step to relieve the feedback?

    1. turn down the volume
    2. remove the hearing aid and reinsert it to ensure it is fit correctly
    3. decrease the high-frequency amplification
    4. change the battery

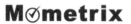

51. The nurse is irrigating a Foley urinary catheter using open intermittent irrigation and has instilled 30 mL of fluid, but the fluid does not drain back after the syringe is removed. What is the next step the nurse should carry out?

    1. turn the client onto the side facing the nurse
    2. notify the physician
    3. aspirate the fluid with the syringe
    4. instill 30 mL more fluid and then check for drainage

52. Following a stroke, a client has impaired swallowing and is unable to feed himself. What is the best position to place the client in when preparing to assist him with meals?

    1. semi-Fowler's, head in midline position, and chin tilted upward
    2. supine position, head in midline, and chin tilted downward
    3. upright position, head in midline, and chin tilted downward
    4. upright position, head in midline, and chin tilted upward

53. A client with chronic obstructive pulmonary disease (COPD) feels breathless despite oxygen administration and bronchodilators. Which of the following positions should the nurse place the client in to best relieve breathlessness?

    1. semi-Fowler's, at 30°
    2. high Fowler's, upright at 90°
    3. semi-Fowler's, at 45°
    4. leaning forward at 30° to 40°

54. A client with moderately advanced dementia is frequently incontinent of urine. Which scheduled urination regimen is most appropriate for this client?

    1. bladder training
    2. timed voiding
    3. patterned urge response toileting
    4. prompted voiding

55. The nurse is caring for a client with a spinal cord injury at T3, and the client is showing signs and symptoms of autonomic dysreflexia. The client uses intermittent clean catheterization and is due for scheduled catheterization.

    I. Loosen any constrictive clothing.
    II. Check the bladder and catheterize the client.
    III. Check for fecal impaction.
    IV. Check the blood pressure (BP) and pulse.
    V. Check the BP and administer a rapid-acting antihypertensive agent if the systolic BP is ≥150 mm Hg.

Place the interventions (in Roman numerals) in the correct order from first to last.

    1. (First) _____
    2. (Second) _____
    3. (Third) _____
    4. (Fourth) _____
    5. (Fifth) _____

56. Which of the following findings place a client at a high risk for suicide? Select all that apply.

    1. older age

    2. previous violent suicide attempt (using a knife or gun)

    3. previous suicide attempt at an isolated site

    4. history of depression 10 years previously

    5. current history of mental illness and disordered thinking

57. A client hospitalized for cocaine overdose has removed his intravenous line and is putting on his clothes, stating that he intends to leave the hospital immediately even though he has no discharge order. Which of the following actions is the best response?

    1. tell the client that he is not allowed to leave

    2. call security to detain the client

    3. restrain the client

    4. ask the client to sign the release for leaving against medical advice (AMA)

58. A client has recorded her intake as follows:

8 oz. tea	4 oz. ice cream
4 oz. gelatin dessert	8 oz. water
6 oz. apple juice	6 oz. milk

The nurse must record the fluid intake in milliliters. How many milliliters of fluid intake will the nurse record for this client? *Record your answer using a whole number.*

59. The nurse has recorded a neonate's weight and length in the metric system with the length recorded as 52.5 cm, but the mother asks how much that is in inches. How many inches are equal to 52.5 cm? *Record your answer using a whole number.*

60. A 16-year-old female client is hospitalized for anorexia nervosa. Which of the following behaviors should the nurse report to the physician? Select all that apply.

    1. the client walks about the grounds with her friend each morning

    2. the client jogs in place for extended periods of time three or four times daily

    3. the client complains daily about constipation, demanding laxatives

    4. the client drinks one to two liters of water daily

    5. the client states that she doesn't need to be in the hospital and refuses to leave her room or interact with other clients

61. The nurse is preparing a client for a mastectomy for treatment of breast cancer. Which of the following should the nurse include in the preoperative teaching? Select all that apply.

    1. wound care

    2. lymphedema control

    3. deep-breathing and coughing exercises

    4. preoperative restrictions on eating and drinking

    5. instruction regarding use of patient-controlled analgesia (PCA)

62. The nurse is caring for a three-year-old child with sickle cell anemia. The nurse expects that the child will receive which of the following treatments routinely as prophylaxis to prevent complications? Select all that apply.

    1. penicillin
    2. blood transfusions
    3. hydroxyurea
    4. opioids
    5. oxygen therapy

63. A client is treated in the emergency department for rape, and a rape kit is completed. The client remains calm, staring at the wall, and she does not appear upset or traumatized, stating repeatedly that she is "fine." Based on these observations, the nurse believes which of the following?

    1. the client is in a state of denial
    2. the client is lying about the rape
    3. the client is in shock
    4. the client suffered a head injury during the rape

64. A client arrives at the emergency department with a sliver of metal penetrating his right eye, resulting from a work injury. Which of the following initial actions does the nurse anticipate?

    1. cover the affected eye with patch
    2. irrigate the affected eye
    3. remove the penetrating object with forceps
    4. request consultation with an ophthalmologist

65. The team leader has asked the nurse to change the tracheostomy tube on a client, but the nurse has never done this procedure before. Which of the following is the correct action for the nurse to take?

    1. ask another nurse on the team to assist with the procedure
    2. look up the procedure in the procedure manual before attempting it
    3. ask the team leader for assistance with the procedure
    4. use a smartphone to access a YouTube video showing how to do the procedure

66. The nurse should advise parents that, because of the danger of choking, children up to three years of age should not be fed which of the following foods? Select all that apply.

    1. beef
    2. peanuts
    3. popcorn
    4. round hard candies
    5. hot dogs
    6. cooked carrots

67. A client with fourth-stage cancer of the colon tells the nurse that he has opted to receive no treatment, even though his life may be prolonged with surgery and chemotherapy, because he feels that the emotional and financial costs to himself and to his family are too high. Which of the following responses is most appropriate for the nurse to make?

    1. "I hope you will reconsider."
    2. "I'm sure your family would rather bear the emotional and financial costs than to lose you."
    3. "The palliative care and hospice program can help you with comfort measures, such as pain control."
    4. "I think you've made the right decision."

68. A client tells the nurse, "I was awake half the night suffering!" Which of the following responses demonstrates therapeutic communication?

    1. "Your pain is not well controlled."
    2. "You should have asked for more pain medication."
    3. "Why didn't you call the nurse?"
    4. "You poor thing. I'm so sorry."

69. Which pain assessment tool is the most appropriate to use with an adolescent?

    1. face, legs, activity, cry, consolability (FLACC) scale
    2. Wong–Baker FACES pain rating scale
    3. Children's Hospital of Eastern Ontario Pain Scale (CHEOPS)
    4. one-to-ten scale

70. The nurse is assessing an elderly client with severe nausea and vomiting for dehydration. Which of the following signs and symptoms are indicative of dehydration? Select all that apply.

    1. urinary specific gravity of 1.006
    2. decrease in hemoglobin and hematocrit
    3. poor skin turgor
    4. dry mucous membranes
    5. decreased thirst
    6. weakness and dizziness

71. A 72-year-old client with osteoarthritis tells the nurse she has not been bathing regularly because standing in the shower is difficult. Which of the following suggestions by the nurse is the most appropriate?

    1. referral to a home health agency for assistance in bathing
    2. use of a shower chair
    3. use of microwavable disposable cloths for sponge baths
    4. referral to an occupational therapist

72. A 76-year-old client became a widow 10 years previously, but she speaks about her husband almost constantly, visits his grave daily, cries daily, and appears unable to make decisions or care for herself because of grief. How would the nurse best describe the client's grieving?

    1. prolonged
    2. normal
    3. delayed
    4. distorted

73. The nurse is monitoring a woman in labor. During which stage of labor does the nurse expect that the woman will become fully dilated (10 cm)?

    1. first stage
    2. second stage
    3. third stage
    4. fourth stage

74. A client involved in a motorcycle accident has a complete spinal cord injury at level C8. Which of the following functional abilities would the nurse expect to observe?

    1. requires an electric wheelchair with breath or head controls and assistance with all activities of daily living (ADLs)
    2. able to use a manual wheelchair on level surfaces but not all surfaces and may shave, brush hair, and is able to feed herself with adaptive equipment
    3. able to use a manual wheelchair on most surfaces, and she is independent in transferring and personal care
    4. requires an electric wheelchair with hand controls, and she is able to feed herself with adaptive equipment

75. A client receiving total parenteral nutrition (TPN) is exhibiting lethargy and changes in mental status as well as asterixis (flapping tremors of the hands). Which of the following interventions does the nurse anticipate?

    1. increase the dextrose concentration of the formula
    2. decrease the dextrose concentration of the formula
    3. decrease the protein concentration of the formula
    4. increase lipid intake

76. Which of the following is an indication of primary graft dysfunction in a lung transplant recipient?

    1. frequent oxygen desaturation
    2. chest pressure
    3. fever
    4. cough

77. Which of the following positions may result in blood pooling in the extremities, decreased blood pressure (BP) and cardiac output, increased respiratory effort, decreased lung compliance, and decreased cerebral circulation?

    1. trendelenburg
    2. right side-lying
    3. supine
    4. prone

78. The nurse is caring for a dying client. Which of the following symptoms indicate that death will occur within a few days? Select all that apply.

    1. the client is increasingly lethargic and disoriented
    2. the client has increasing dysphagia
    3. the client is extremely weak, gaunt, and pale
    4. the client is drinking only four or five ounces of water at a time
    5. the client is incontinent of a small amount of concentrated urine
    6. the client has a decreased cardiac rate

79. According to federal law, if a client dies in a hospital setting, which of the following must be done by the staff?

1. the coroner must be notified
2. the family decision maker must be asked about organ donation
3. the family must be provided information about funeral regulations
4. the Social Security Administration must be notified

80. The nurse is opening a sterile dressing pack to change the dressing on a client's abdominal wound. Which of the following actions will contaminate the contents of the pack?

1. the nurse holds the sterile dressing below waist level when transferring it to the sterile drape
2. the nurse holds the package in his nondominant hand while peeling the wrapper over the nondominant hand with his other hand
3. the nurse positions the bottom half of the sterile drape over the top half of the work surface before placing the top half of the drape over the bottom half of the work surface
4. the nurse opens the outermost flap of the sterile kit away from his body

81. A client with deficiency of coagulation factors because of liver disease is to receive 10 mL of fresh frozen plasma per kg of body weight. The client's weight is 183 lb (83 kg). How many milliliters of FFP should the client receive? Record your answer using a whole number.

_____ milliliters.

82. If a patient was involved in a motorcycle accident and is nonresponsive and on a ventilator, which of the following tests must be performed to diagnose brain death prior to organ donation? Select all that apply.

1. two electroencephalograms (EEGs) taken 12 to 24 hours apart
2. two electrocardiograms (ECGs) taken 12 to 24 hours apart
3. testing of brainstem reflexes
4. apnea testing
5. transcranial Doppler ultrasonography

83. Although the sister of a client with end-stage kidney disease has stated she will donate a kidney to her brother, she actually does not want to do so even though testing shows she is a good match. However, she does not want her brother or family to know that she has refused to donate a kidney. If the client asks if his sister is honest about not being a match, which of the following is the most appropriate response?

1. "I don't believe she was a match."
2. "You should ask your sister."
3. "I don't know the answer to that question."
4. "You should discuss that with your doctor."

84. A client with end-stage liver disease is to be discharged from the acute care hospital to his home; however, the client has stated he does not want hospice and that his family will care for him. Which of the following is the most appropriate response?

1. tell the client she is placing too large a burden on family
2. advise the client that she is making a mistake
3. insist the client reconsider and accept hospice care
4. provide information about the benefits of hospice

85. Which of the following interventions are indicated as part of post-mortem care? Select all that apply.

1. position limbs in proper alignment
2. dress the client in burial clothing
3. place dentures in the mouth
4. cleanse the body gently as necessary
5. tape the eyes closed or place weighted items on the eyelids

86. In the normal electrocardiogram (ECG) complex, the QRS complex represents which of the following?

1. ventricular repolarization
2. AV mode depolarization
3. atrial depolarization
4. ventricular depolarization

87. A client has had a ventricular pacemaker implanted, but he has lethargy, headache, pain in the jaw, breathlessness, and anxiety. On examination, the nurse notes pulsations evident in the neck and the abdomen. Which of the following is the most likely reason for the client's symptoms?

1. client is having a panic attack
2. client is experiencing pacemaker syndrome
3. client is having a myocardial infarction
4. client is experiencing pacemaker-mediated tachycardia

88. If a client is to undergo gastric lavage after ingesting poison, what position should the nurse place the client in for the procedure?

1. semi-Fowler's position with head elevated to 30 to 40 degrees
2. upright position with head elevated to 80 to 90 degrees
3. trendelenburg position with the client supine
4. left lateral position with head lowered 15 degrees

89. A client has been admitted through the emergency department after an acute episode of GI hemorrhage. The client's hemoglobin is 6.1 and hematocrit is 18.3. The client is a Jehovah's Witness and has refused transfusions even though his hemoglobin and hematocrit are still falling; the physician has advised him that he might die without transfusions. Which of the following is the most appropriate response for the nurse?

1. provide supportive care and respect the client's right to refuse treatment
2. urge the client to consider his family and reconsider his decision
3. tell the client that his decision is unreasonable
4. ask the client's family members to reason with the client

90. A client with severe diarrhea, nausea, and vomiting has become increasingly lethargic and weak with tingling in the hands and feet, muscle cramps and tetany, hypotension, and dysrhythmias with ECG abnormalities that include PVCs and flattened T waves. Based on these signs and symptoms, which of the following electrolyte imbalances should the nurse suspect?

1. hypokalemia
2. hyperkalemia
3. hyponatremia
4. hypernatremia

91. Which of the following orders utilize correct abbreviations? Select all that apply.

1. MS 10.0 mg SC stat
2. DSS Q.D.
3. Levothyroxine 0.112 mg daily
4. Acetaminophen 650 mg at HS
5. TCN 500 mg BID

92. The unit supervisor assigns a nurse to three clients for primary care, but the nurse discovers that one of the clients is a close neighbor and casual friend. Which of the following is the most appropriate action?

1. care for the patient as assigned
2. ask the client if the assignment is acceptable
3. informally ask another nurse to trade clients
4. ask the supervisor to reassign the client

93. Which of the following are HIPAA violations? Select all that apply.

1. the nurse shares information about the client with the client's sister
2. the nurse allows another nurse to "shoulder surf" the client's EHR
3. the nurse accesses the history and physical of a client assigned to the nurse
4. the nurse discusses the client's concerns about treatment with the physician
5. the nurse tells the client's physician that the client expressed suicidal ideation

94. The nurse is assigned as team leader for an LVN and 2 CNAs. The nurse must delegate a number of different tasks:

- dressing change on a foot ulcer
- insertion of a Foley catheter
- enema as prep for a radiological procedure
- bed baths for four clients
- checking routine vital signs

Which task(s) should the nurse assign to the LVN?

1. dressing change only
2. dressing change and insertion of a Foley catheter
3. dressing change and enema
4. dressing change, enema, and insertion of Foley catheter

95. A client has been exploring different types of complementary therapies. Which of the following statements by the client indicate a need for education? Select all that apply.

    1. "I don't need to worry about taking herbs because they're natural."
    2. "Acupuncture may help to relieve back pain."
    3. "Homeopathic medicine is better for infections than antibiotics."
    4. "Relaxation exercises can help to reduce anxiety."
    5. "I should check with the doctor before taking herbal preparations."
    6. "I've heard that there is an herbal cure for cancer in Mexico."

96. If a client has expressed a desire to quit smoking and asks the nurse for advice, what is the first step that the nurse should suggest the client take?

    1. throw away cigarettes
    2. ask family members to provide support
    3. make a quit plan
    4. sign a contract agreeing to quit

97. Which of the following are required components of an informed consent? Select all that apply.

    1. duration of procedure
    2. alternative options
    3. nature and reason for procedure
    4. risks and benefits
    5. explanation of diagnosis

98. The nurse is concerned that the procedures commonly used for wound care are outdated and wants to move toward a more evidence-based approach. Which of the following is the best place to begin to gather information?

    1. survey physicians
    2. search medical databases
    3. look through books in the medical library
    4. contact healthcare providers specializing in wound care

99. Following a client's death, the nurse helps the client's daughter reposition the client, and the daughter insists that she heard the client breathe as the client was moved. Which of the following is the best response?

    1. tell the daughter she was mistaken about hearing respirations
    2. listen to the client's lungs for signs of respirations to reassure the daughter
    3. explain that trapped air escaped from the lungs when the client was moved
    4. tell the daughter that the sound she heard was normal after death

100. A client is admitted for treatment of a myocardial infarction but insists on leaving against medical advice (AMA). The nurse has attempted to reach the physician, who has not responded. Which of the following measures should the nurse take? Select all that apply.

    1. advise the client of health risks of leaving before treatment is completed
    2. assess the client's mental status and ability to make decisions
    3. ask the client to sign an AMA form
    4. arrange for follow-up by phone or return visit
    5. advise the client that he cannot leave until the physician arrives

101. A physician has telephoned a number of orders for a client who has developed a fever and chills. Which of the following is the correct procedure when taking telephone orders?

1. write the orders directly into the client's record as given
2. write the orders in their entirety and then read back and confirm
3. repeat each order one at a time and ask for confirmation for each before proceeding
4. insist the physician email or fax a copy of the orders for confirmation

102. An 11-year-old child with autism spectrum disorder is hospitalized but is frequently extremely agitated, refusing to take medications and screaming and hitting his head against the bed headboard, when the parents are not present. Which of the following is likely the most effective method of controlling the child's behavior?

1. ask the parents for advice
2. ask the physician for a sedative
3. place the child in restraints
4. ask a physician for a psychiatric referral

103. An elderly client hospitalized for a stroke from a long-term care facility has a large diamond ring that is very loose and has fallen off of the client's finger twice. The nurse is concerned that the ring will be lost or stolen, especially since the client has expressive aphasia. Which of the following is the best course of action?

1. remove the ring and secure according to hospital policy
2. remove the ring and send it home with the client's caregiver
3. leave the ring in place and tape it to the finger
4. leave the ring in place and take no further action

104. The physician has written an order for the nurse to remove a client's running sutures since the incision is well healed. The running suture line has 8 stitches (including the knotted stitches at the ends). When the suture removal is completed, how many individual pieces of suture should the nurse have removed?

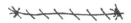

1. one
2. two
3. three
4. eight

105. A patient underwent a fiberoptic bronchoscopy for right lung biopsy under conscious sedation, but within a few minutes of being sent to the recovery room, the client shows increasing signs of dyspnea and, although groggy, has ipsilateral chest pain. The pulse rate increases from 82 to 100, and the client is slightly hypotensive and coughing. Which of the following should the nurse suspect?

1. heart attack
2. pulmonary edema
3. pneumothorax or bleeding
4. pulmonary embolism

106. If monitoring a client's control of diabetes, which of the following sources of information is the most reliable?

  1. serum glucose level
  2. HbA1c
  3. client's food and exercise log
  4. client's diet/exercise log

107. If a client with bipolar disorder is exhibiting disturbed thought processes as evidenced by delusional thinking, which of the following is the most appropriate response?

  1. "You are wrong about what you are thinking."
  2. "Try to think about this logically, and you'll see what you believe is impossible."
  3. "I understand you believe this, but I don't see evidence that this is true."
  4. "Look around. You are the only person who believes this!"

108. When doing nasotracheal suctioning, during which of the following should the catheter be inserted?

  1. inhalation
  2. exhalation
  3. swallowing
  4. coughing

109. When changing an colostomy appliance, with which of the following should the skin about the stoma be cleansed after the pouch is removed?

  1. soap and water
  2. alcohol swabs
  3. tap water
  4. baby wipes

110. A client with a long history of alcohol abuse has been hospitalized with diabetic complications. On the seventh day of hospitalization and 7 days after the last drink, the client begins to hallucinate and becomes increasingly agitated and confused. The client's blood pressure and pulse are both increasing, and the client is perspiring profusely and temperature has elevated to 38°C. Based on this clinical profile, which of the following complications should the nurse consider?

  1. major withdrawal
  2. minor withdrawal
  3. withdrawal seizures
  4. delirium tremens

111. A 7-month-old infant with community-acquired pneumonia (*H. influenzae*) has received a loading dose of azithromycin oral suspension at dosage of 10 mg/kg of body weight on day 1 in the emergency department and is now to receive 5 mg/kg per day on days 2 through 5 (to a maximum of 250 mg per day). The infant's weight is 16.5 lb. How many milligrams should the infant receive on days 2 to 5? Record your answer using a number with one decimal point.

  _____ milligrams.

112. If the nurse examining the blisters of a client in the active phase of herpes zoster (shingles) has direct contact with bare hands to the fluid in some of the blisters, the nurse may be at risk of developing which of the following?

1. herpes zoster (shingles)
2. varicella zoster virus (chickenpox)
3. viral meningitis
4. there is no risk of transmission

113. A new mother is concerned that her neonate is having periods of apnea. What duration of apnea is of concern in the neonate?

1. all periods of apnea
2. 2-3 seconds
3. 6 to 8 seconds
4. >15 to 20 seconds

114. A client who is 2 months pregnant states that she has never received a measles vaccination and was exposed to a child with measles 14 days earlier. The client asks the nurse if she is still at risk of developing measles. Which of the following is the most accurate information?

1. the client is no longer at risk
2. the client is at risk for another 2 days
3. the client is at risk for another 7 days
4. the client is at risk for another 14 days

115. If a client is walking in the hall and falls to the floor with a tonic-clonic seizure, which of the following actions by the nurse is the most appropriate. Select all that apply.

1. turn client to one side with head slightly flexed forward
2. restrain the client to prevent injury
3. insert a padded tongue blade between the teeth if possible
4. support the head with cushioning of some type
5. provide privacy if possible

116. A client brought to the emergency department has been exposed to cold temperatures, and his core body temperature is 34°C. Which of the following rewarming techniques is most indicated?

1. cardiopulmonary bypass
2. warm IV fluid administration
3. warm peritoneal lavage
4. forced air warm blankets

117. The nurse is examining a client's incision following a radical nephrectomy. Which of the following signs or symptoms may be most indicative of infection? Select all that apply.

1. slight serosanguineous discharge is evident on the dressing
2. tissue about incision is moderately edematous and increasingly erythematous
3. the dressing that has covered the incision has a foul odor
4. the client has pain in the incisional area
5. there is purulent discharge from the wound

118. Which of the following dressing types is most appropriate for a stage II pressure ulcer with moderate amounts of exudate?

1. NS on gauze (wet-to-dry)
2. transparent film
3. hydrocolloid
4. hydrogel

119. A client with kidney failure is considering continuous ambulatory peritoneal dialysis (CAPD). The client asks the nurse for information about CAPD. Which of the following information should the nurse include? Select all that apply.

1. exchanges are usually done with about 2 L of dialysate
2. most clients do 4 to 5 exchanges in a 24-hour period.
3. each exchange takes 30 to 40 minutes
4. an exchange is a clean rather than sterile procedure
5. exchanges at night involve a longer period of retention

120. A client is undergoing negative pressure wound therapy (NPWT). Which of the following tasks associated with NPWT can be delegated to unlicensed assistive personnel (UAP)? Select all that apply.

1. disconnect NPWT unit and remove dressings
2. apply new dressings and connect the NPWT unit
3. report changes in client's comfort level
4. monitor tubing to prevent displacement when turning client
5. assess condition of the wound

Answer Key and Explanations for Test #2

1. 1: Confused clients with Alzheimer's disease should be placed in a private room to minimize disturbances to other clients. The client should be near the nursing station and within the nurses' line of sight so a close watch can be kept over the client. Restraints should be avoided if at all possible because they often cause clients to become more agitated. Clients who are confused and trying to climb out of bed may require a sitter during hospitalization.

2. 4: The most effective method of reducing the spread of nosocomial infections, such as *Clostridium difficile*, is by practicing a thorough, consistent handwashing routine. The hands may be routinely decontaminated with alcohol-based hand rubs or antimicrobial soap and water. If the hands are visibly dirty or contaminated with body fluids (feces, urine, blood, or sputum), then they should be washed under running water with nonantimicrobial soap and water or antimicrobial soap and water. The hands should be decontaminated before and after direct contact with clients and before and after donning gloves.

3. 1, 4, and 5: Research has shown that acupuncture and massage may help to reduce chronic lower back pain. Acupuncture is a part of traditional Chinese medicine in which tiny needles are inserted into acupoints and left in place for 30 to 60 minutes to balance the vital energy. Massage helps to relax the muscles and relieve discomfort. Visualization and relaxation can benefit almost all clients because they can help to reduce anxiety and relax tense muscles. There is no evidence that aromatherapy or homeopathy is effective in reducing chronic lower back pain.

4. 2: Following the death of a client, rigor mortis usually begins within two to four hours because adenosine triphosphate (ATP), which is necessary to relax muscles, is no longer synthesized, so muscles contract. It's important to position the client before rigor mortis begins. This includes closing the eyes, placing dentures in the mouth, closing the jaw (using a rolled towel to keep the mouth closed), positioning the hands, and positioning the body in correct alignment.

5. Correct order:

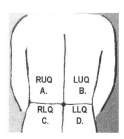

1. (RUQ) III. Liver and gallbladder.
2. (LUQ) II. Spleen.
3. (RLQ) I. Cecum and appendix.
4. (LLQ) IV. Sigmoid colon.

6. One percent (1%) solution: Epinephrine 1:100 means that there is 1 part medication to 100 parts diluent. Calculation:

1/100 = 0.01.
0.01 × 100 = 1%.

63

7. 3: When administering total parenteral nutrition (TPN), the filters, tubing, and solution should be changed every 24 hours. Aseptic technique must be maintained to avoid infection, vital signs (VS) should be monitored every 4 hours, and weight should be checked daily. Laboratory testing is usually done at least every three days until the client stabilizes and then at least one time weekly. Cloudiness in the formula indicates contamination, so any cloudy solution should be immediately discarded. Micropore filters are used for solutions without fat emulsion, and 0.1-micron filters are used for solutions with fat emulsion.

8. 1: The Tensilon (edrophonium chloride) test is used to diagnose myasthenia gravis. Tensilon is an anticholinesterase medication used to increase levels of acetylcholine at the myoneural junctions to relieve symptoms. For the test, the patient is given an injection of Tensilon. If the symptoms are relieved, then the test is positive for myasthenia gravis. If the symptoms remain the same or worsen, then the test is negative. Tensilon is also used to determine if the client is under- or overmedicated with anticholinesterase.

9. 4: The nurse should apply an earlobe oximeter. A digit pulse oximeter should be avoided if the client has tremors or if he is likely to move his hand frequently. The skin should be clean and dry when the oximeter is applied. If using a digit oximeter, a client should not have artificial nails or wear colored nail polish because these may interfere with readings. If a client is severely obese, the clip on the oximeter may not stay in place, so a disposable (single-use) sensor pad may be necessary.

10. 3: Edema is a common problem related to burns, so the nurse must check peripheral pulses frequently (at least every two hours) and keep the extremities elevated on two pillows. If the pulses become diminished, the first step is to loosen the dressings and recheck the pulses to determine if the dressings are restricting blood flow. Burns are often treated with topical agents and several layers of dressings, which should be applied on the lower extremities distally to proximally.

11. 2: The nurse should immediately notify the radiation department and make no attempt to touch or move the radiation source. Nurses caring for the client should minimize their time in the room and maximize the distance from the source of radiation (such as standing at the door instead of next to the bed to speak with the client). Although the client should have all necessary care, the nurse must avoid excessive exposure to radiation and may be required to wear appropriate shielding. Nurses who are pregnant should not be involved in care of clients undergoing radiation therapy.

12. 1, 2, 4, and 5: Clients need adaptive equipment to allow them to be independent in their own care and to prevent injury to the hip during the healing process. Equipment that is considered to be necessary on discharge includes a walker, an elevated toilet seat, a reacher/grabber to pick things up, and a sock aid to assist the client to dress. Most clients should not need a wheelchair after discharge unless they have comorbidities. Although some clients may be ready to use a cane on discharge, most are still dependent on walkers, which provide better stability.

13. 4: The best solution to an influx of clients during an emergency situation is to carry out early discharge for low-risk, noncritical clients. Often, elective procedures, such as ambulatory surgeries and testing, are canceled and rescheduled. Clients may be sent home with home health care or, in some cases, transferred to other facilities, such as convalescent hospitals. Each facility should have a disaster plan in place that outlines the steps to take in an emergency.

14. 1, 2, and 4: Findings consistent with end-stage renal disease (ESRD) include the following:

- Decreased creatinine clearance: Decreases as glomerular filtration rate decreases, while the serum creatinine and blood urea nitrogen (BUN) levels increase.
- Metabolic acidosis: Results from a decreased ability of the kidneys to excrete ammonia and reabsorb sodium bicarbonate.
- Anemia: Results from inadequate production of erythropoietin by the kidneys.
- Fluid retention related to hypernatremia: Increases the risk of heart failure and edema.
- Hyperphosphatemia and hypocalcemia: The kidneys cannot adequately filter out phosphorus, so hyperphosphatemia results in hypocalcemia because of a reciprocal relationship.

15. 2: "The company is exempt from the provisions of the ADA because of its size" is the correct response because small businesses employing 15 or fewer employees are not required to comply with the provisions of the ADA even though cancer is considered to be a disability. However, the client should be encouraged to discuss her needs with her employer because some may be willing to make reasonable accommodations. The ADA (1990) is intended to protect persons with disabilities against discrimination. The ADA was amended in 2008.

16. 4: The apical pulse is assessed at the fifth left intercostal space at the midclavicular line, which is the point of maximal impulse. The nurse first locates the sternal notch, and from there the second intercostal space and then moves her fingers lightly down the side of the sternum to the fifth intercostal space and over to the midclavicular line. The nurse should be able to auscultate the S1 and S2 normal heart sounds at this point.

17. 2: When a mother has an autosomal-dominant gene, each child has a 50% chance of inheriting the gene. However, because inheritance is a random process, this does not mean that 50% will actually inherit the gene. In fact, all children or no children may inherit. Humans should have 23 pairs of chromosomes: Pairs 1 to 22 are autosomal, and pair 23 is sex with XX for female and XY for male.

N = normal gene, and D = dominant mutated gene.

	N	**D**
N	N N	N D (mutation)
N	N N	N D (mutation)

18. 1: Oral steroids should never be abruptly discontinued and replaced by inhaled steroids because the inhaled steroids alone produce lower plasma levels than do oral preparations. Tapering allows the adrenal glands to recover and function properly. The prednisone dosage should be tapered while the inhaled steroid is introduced to avoid exacerbation of the client's COPD. Clients who have been on oral steroids for extended periods of time may have difficulty with the transition to inhaled steroids and must be monitored carefully.

19. 1, 4, 5, and 6: Parkinson's disease is related to deficiency of the neurotransmitter dopamine. Signs and symptoms include resting tremor (usually unilateral initially of the upper extremity, but it may affect the foot or face), rigidity, bradykinesia, postural instability, dysphagia, and flat affect. Clients with Parkinson's disease often walk leaning forward and with a short, shuffling gait with a reduced arm swing. Speech is often slow and slightly slurred with a monotonous tone. Many clients exhibit micrographia (small, illegible writing).

20. 4: The correct dosage in grams is 3 g piperacillin/0.375 g tazobactam. Calculation:

30 (weight in kg) × 100 (mg piperacillin) = 3000 mg.
30 (weight in kg) × 12.5 (mg tazobactam) = 375 mg.

To convert milligrams to grams:

3000/1000 = 3 g piperacillin.
375/1,000 = 0.375 g tazobactam.

21. 1 and 4: The expected outcomes should relate specifically to the nursing diagnosis (rather than the clinical diagnosis) and interventions:
- Nursing diagnosis: Chronic low self-esteem.
- Intervention 1: Self-esteem enhancement—Help the client identify and review negative perceptions of self. Encourage him to take an active role in his treatment planning.
- Intervention 2: Self-awareness enhancement—Help the client identify personal positive beliefs and characteristics as well as self-limiting behaviors.
- Expected outcomes: The client is able to use positive self-talk to interrupt negative thinking. He is able to use positive coping behaviors to improve his functioning.

22. 110 mg. Calculation:

22 (kg of weight) × 15 (mg of gabapentin) = 330 mg.

This is the total dosage, but it is to be given in three divided doses:

330/3 = 110 mg per dose.

23. 1: The client should be advised to avoid sunbathing because tetracycline causes photosensitivity, which can occur immediately upon exposure or sometime after exposure to sunlight. Tetracycline should be taken with a full glass of water one hour before or two hours after meals. Clients should be cautioned that milk, other dairy products, and iron products reduce the absorption of tetracycline, so they should not be taken within two hours of the drug dosing. Tetracycline should not be given to children younger than eight years of age.

24. 2, 4, 5, and 6: Addisonian crisis is an acute episode of adrenal insufficiency that is life threatening and precipitated by a stressor, such as gastrointestinal infection, fever, or surgery. Addisonian crisis may be misdiagnosed as acute abdomen because clients may present with nausea and severe abdominal pain. Shock, with hypotension and pallor, is common, and clients may exhibit tachycardia, confusion, and restlessness. Because temperature regulation is impaired, clients may exhibit hypothermia or hyperthermia. Suspected Addisonian crisis must be treated immediately because clients may die while awaiting test results.

25. 22 mL. Calculation:

55 (kg of weight) × 2 (mg of metoclopramide HCl) = 110 mg.

The medication is provided with 5 mg per mL:

110 (mg)/5 (mg per mL) = 22 mL of medication.

26. 3: Cholecystitis may result in severe episodes of pain in the right upper quadrant of the abdomen, often lasting two to six hours, and sometimes radiating to the back. Clients may also experience indigestion, nausea and vomiting, and clay-colored stools if the bile duct is blocked. In severe cases, jaundice may be evident. Cholecystitis may result from calculi or pancreatitis and is most common in overweight females ages 20 to 40, but it also may occur in women who are pregnant.

27. 4: The hand is used for palpation, but different parts of the hand are sensitive to different things. The dorsum (back surface) of the hand is most sensitive to variations in skin temperature, such as may occur during an infection or fever. The palm of the hand is used to detect vibrations, such as on the chest wall. The fingertips are very sensitive to shape and texture and are also used to assess pulsations, such as the radial and carotid pulses.

28. 1: The statement "She purposely hides her belongings from me" suggests that the daughter-in-law believes that the client's behavior is intentional rather than related to confusion. This is a common misconception. Caregivers may blame cognitively impaired clients for their behavior and become angry when the behavior persists. Putting things in the wrong place and forgetting their placement are typical behaviors for clients with Alzheimer's disease. The nurse needs to review behaviors associated with Alzheimer's diseases and discuss coping strategies.

29. 4: After medication is injected into the port of an intravenous bag, it will tend to pool in the lower part of the bag, so the nurse should gently shake the bag to distribute the medication more evenly throughout the solution. The infusion bag must be labeled according to facility policy, usually with the patient's name, room number, name of the medication, date and time the medication is mixed, date and time the infusion is started, and the initials of the nurse administering the infusion.

30. 3: The nurse should instruct the client to open her mouth and hold the inhaler one to two inches in front of her mouth (about two finger widths). The client should exhale and then inhale deeply for 5 seconds while pressing down on the inhaler to release a dose of medication. After inhaling the medication, the client should hold her breath for about 10 seconds and then exhale slowly through pursed lips. Children and those who have difficulty managing the procedure should use spacers.

31. 1: Clients must avoid placing direct sources of heat, such as a heating pad, over a fentanyl patch because this action increases the rate of absorption and may cause the client to have an overdose. Clients are allowed to bathe or shower wearing the patch, but this may cause the patch to loosen, so clients may cover the patch with plastic wrap taped in place over the patch while bathing if this tends to occur. A patch should be disposed of by rolling it and flushing it down the toilet because some medication will remain in the patch.

32. 4: *N*-acetylcysteine is the antidote for acetaminophen overdose. Acetaminophen toxicity occurs with a single dose of greater than 140 mg/kg of body weight or with greater than 7.5 g in 24 hours. The antidote is given for serum levels greater than 150. It is most effective if given with 8 hours of ingestion. *N*-acetylcysteine is given at the rate of 140 mg/kg initially and repeated with 70 mg/kg every 4 hours for 17 additional doses, either by mouth or intravenously.

33. 18 mL. Calculation:

80 (mg)/15 (ml) = 96 (mg)/x (ml)
80 × x = 80x
15 × 96 = 1,440
80x = 1,440
8x = 144
144/8 = 18 mL

34. 2: The nurse should assist the client into a position of comfort on the floor and use a mechanical lift to raise the client. There is no other lift that will raise the client and not pose a risk of injury to the nurse or those assisting. If the client is fairly mobile and strong, he may be assisted into a four-point position on his knees, and a chair is placed next to him so he can raise himself with minimal assistance.

35. 3: The nurse should telephone the physician to question the dosage and should be prepared to tell the physician the client's weight in kilograms and the recommended dosage. In some cases, the physician may have a valid reason for exceeding the usual dosage, but the staff should be aware of the reasons. It is the nurse's responsibility to ensure that the five rights of medication administration are adhered to: right client, right drug, right dose, right route, and right time.

36. 1, 3, 4, and 5: Most infant abductors are female, approximately age 30, and overweight. They rarely have a criminal record and may appear quite normal, although they may be emotionally immature and behave impulsively. Abductors often visit the site of abduction in advance and may ask many questions about procedures and nursery policies and may try to become friendly with staff and parents to gain information and trust. Abductors often seek to replace a child they have lost or to compensate for their inability to have children.

37. 2: The nurse is participating in community health education by providing alcohol-based cleansers and also by educating the public about methods to prevent the flu. Community health education may be formal, with classes scheduled on a number of different health topics, or informal, such as answering questions about health matters and setting an example for others in the community. The nurse often serves as a resource person for others with questions about health matters.

38. 3: Extended family: Multigenerational families or shared households with parents, friends, or other family members, such as aunts and uncles. Nuclear family: The traditional family with mother, father, and children. Generally, the husband is the breadwinner in this model and the mother remains at home to care for the children. Coparenting: Custody is shared between two families, such as with a divorce custody agreements. Extended kin network: Two nuclear families live together or near each other and share goods and services, such as childcare.

39. 250 minutes. Calculation:

15 (drops)/ 1 (minute) × 1 (ml)/15 (drops).
15 × 1 = 15.
15 × 1 = 15.
15/15 = 1 ml/min.
250 (ml) × 1 (ml/min) = 250 minutes.

40. 1, 3, and 4: The nurse cannot delegate assessment regarding the initial need for restraints, the ongoing need, or the type of restraint. However, unlicensed assistive personnel may apply restraints if they have been trained to do so; position clients while they are in restraints; check restraints for correct placement; and provide any supportive care, such as toileting and providing fluids and skin care under the guidance of the nurse, who should provide clear instructions regarding how long the restraints are to be in place and how frequently the client should be turned or what other care should be provided.

41. 1: The best solution to dealing with a client's discomfort is to acknowledge the discomfort in a supportive manner: "I can see that these questions are making you uncomfortable because it's difficult for most people to talk about personal issues." Joking about the client's discomfort or ignoring it altogether shows a lack of respect for the client's feelings, and stopping the questions is not a good solution because the information may be important for providing a full understanding of the client and his health issues.

42. 4: The best solution to hearing a colleague divulge personal information about a client is to use an "I" statement, which conveys the message that the conversation is inappropriate without being accusing: "I don't feel comfortable violating a client's privacy." If an organization is to maintain an ethical environment, then every member of the staff must be willing to address the issue when it arises so others may understand that gossiping about clients is not acceptable behavior.

43. 2: Although the client may benefit from pain medication prior to treatment because of increased pain associated with administration of chemotherapy and may be less tense if instructed in deep-breathing and relaxation exercises, these are not good solutions for the local discomfort associated with port access. The best solution is to apply EMLA (lidocaine/prilocaine) cream to the port area about 20 to 45 minutes prior to treatment. If receiving chemotherapy as an outpatient, the client can apply the cream and cover the area with plastic wrap before leaving home.

44. 3: If the child is lying prone with a pillow under the abdomen and lower legs and percussion is administered at the base of the scapulae and immediately inferior to the scapulae, the superior segments of the right and left lower lobes are being treated. Chest physiotherapy (CPT) should not be administered on bare skin. Percussion may be done with a CPT cup for very small children and with cupped hands for older children and adults. Vibration is done after the client takes a deep breath and while he exhales.

45. 4: With peritoneal dialysis, a typical exchange cycle takes 30 to 45 minutes and includes three phases: infusion (5 to 10 minutes) of two to three liters of dialysate, dwell time (about 10 minutes), and drainage (10 to 30 minutes). The number of cycles each day is determined on an individual basis. The drainage fluid should be straw-colored or clear. Cloudy drainage may indicate an infection. Blood-tinged drainage may occur shortly after insertion of the abdominal catheter and during menses.

46. 4: If a client with preeclampsia experiences a seizure (indicating eclampsia), the client should be placed in the most protective position for herself and the fetus, the left lateral position. This position decreases the risk that she will aspirate, and it relieves the pressure of the uterus against the vena cava, increasing blood flow to the fetus. The side rails should be raised if the client is in bed, but they should be padded with a blanket or pillows to prevent her from injuring herself.

47. 1, 4, 5, and 6: Any radiation treatments to the abdominal area may result in damage to the cells of the small and large intestines, causing diarrhea. The client should be advised to drink ample (8 to 12 cups) amounts of clear liquid each day and to avoid large meals in favor of five to six small meals daily, which may be better tolerated. Clients may develop rectal irritation, so they should use baby wipes instead of toilet paper or use a squirt bottle with water to cleanse the rectal area. Clients should avoid milk products, fatty foods, gas-producing foods, and fried foods. Imodium® is often prescribed to reduce diarrhea.

48. 2: Total patient care: A nurse is assigned to do all the care of one or two clients. Modified primary care: A nurse is responsible for the same group of clients every day, usually with assistive personnel. Team nursing: A team leader of a group that comprises unlicensed assistive personnel and licensed vocational/practical nurses as well as other registered nurses (RNs) may be responsible for a fairly large group of clients, often ranging from 10 to 20. Functional nursing: Tasks are divided; for example, one nurse may give medications to all clients, and another nurse might do all the dressing changes.

49. 3: Although cooperating, being informed, and evaluating outcomes are all important in continuous quality performance improvement, the nurse's primary responsibility is to actively seek methods to improve performance. The nurse must remain current in the profession; evaluate evidence and seek out best practices; observe methods and outcomes; and look for opportunities to make changes, big and small, that may improve the quality of client care and/or improve the cost-effectiveness of care and return on investment.

50. 2: A frequent cause of acoustic feedback with a hearing aid is incorrect fit, so removing the hearing aid and reinserting it, making sure that it is seated properly in the ear canal may alleviate the problem. If the acoustic feedback persists, then the client may have earwax or the hearing aid may need to be refitted because the fit may be too loose. In some cases, adjusting the high-frequency amplification may reduce acoustic feedback, but it may also decrease the ability to hear speech, so this is usually not a good solution.

51. 1: Because Foley catheters are usually maintained on continuous drainage, the bladder may be essentially empty when it is irrigated, so the small amount of irrigant may pool away from the end of the catheter. Therefore, the best solution if no fluid returns is to turn the client onto the side facing the nurse, being careful to maintain the sterile field. If the irrigant still does not return, then the nurse should gently aspirate using the syringe.

52. 3: The best position for a client with impaired swallowing is upright with the head midline and the chin down (flexed about 75% of the way toward the chest) because this position provides better protection of the airway and decreases the risk of choking and aspirating. The patient may be positioned with the arms on the overbed table with positioning aids used, if necessary, to maintain body alignment. The client should continue to remain in the upright position for at least 30 minutes after the feeding is completed.

53. 4: COPD clients are unable to adequately use accessory muscles of respiration, so leaning forward at 30° to 40° improves the upward movement of the diaphragm, allowing more air to be expelled with each exhalation, and helping to reduce breathlessness. The patient may be positioned with the arms resting on an overbed table if in bed or on the thighs or a small table if sitting in a chair. Many COPD clients sleep sitting up because of increased shortness of breath when they try to recline.

54. 2: Timed voiding: Toileting is carried out on a regularly scheduled basis, usually every two hours during waking hours and one or two times during the night. This is especially useful for those with cognitive impairment. Bladder training: Toileting is scheduled with progressive voiding intervals, but clients must be cognitively aware. Patterned urge response toileting: A form of habit training using an electronic monitoring device. Prompted voiding: Suitable for mild dementia clients, toileting is prompted on a regular schedule for those able to use the toilet independently.

55. Correct order:

1: (First) IV. Check the blood pressure (BP) and pulse.
2: (Second) I. Loosen any constrictive clothing.
3: (Third) II. Check the bladder and catheterize the client.
4: (Fourth) V. Check the BP and administer a rapid-acting antihypertensive agent if the systolic BP is ≥150 mm Hg.
5: (Fifth) III. Check for fecal impaction.

Treatment should always begin by checking vital signs (VS) and loosening clothes and then progressing to assessment of the bladder. If there is no indwelling catheter, the client should be catheterized. If a catheter is in place, it must be checked for patency and irrigated if necessary. The BP should be checked again and an antihypertensive agent administered if the BP remains elevated before checking for fecal impaction.

56. 2, 3, and 4: Clients who have previously attempted violent suicide, such as with a gun or knife; who attempted suicide at an isolated site with little chance of rescue; or who have a current history of mental illness and disordered thinking are at a high risk for suicide. Other risk factors include current severe depression and lack of an adequate social support system. Clients with these risk factors should be monitored carefully. Anyone who has previously attempted suicide in any manner has an increased risk of making another attempt.

57. 4: Unless treatment is court ordered, clients cannot be prevented from leaving the hospital, so telling the client that he cannot leave, calling security, or restraining the client would be to violate his rights to self-determination and could be construed as unlawful imprisonment. The nurse should ask the client to sign the release for leaving against medical advice (AMA) and should follow hospital protocol for such situations. The nurse should ask the client to speak with the physician before leaving.

58. 1,080 mL. Calculation:

8 + 4 + 6 + 4 + 8 + 6 = 36
1 oz. = 30 mL
36 × 30 = 1,080 mL

Note that ice cream and gelatin dessert are considered as liquids when calculating intake and output.

59. 21 inches. Calculation:

1 inch = 2.5 cm.
52.5/2.5 = 21 inches.

60. 2, 3, and 5: Although walking is a healthy exercise, clients with anorexia nervosa often exercise excessively in an effort to lose weight, so jogging in place for extended periods of time at multiple times during the day is a cause for concern. Clients often use laxatives and diuretics to try to induce weight loss, so the nurse should report the client's demand for laxatives. Clients with anorexia frequently experience denial and may become very depressed and withdrawn, and the physician should be notified of this behavior.

61. 3, 4, and 5: Clients should not be overwhelmed with preoperative instructions, so wound care and lymphedema control should be discussed postoperatively. Because lung ventilation is very important after surgery, the client should practice deep-breathing and coughing exercises preoperatively and should know what food and fluid restrictions (such as no fluids for six hours before surgery) must be complied with. Because clients usually return from surgery with patient-controlled analgesia (PCA) in place, instructions about its use should occur preoperatively when the client is more alert and not yet in pain.

62. 1 and 3: Prophylaxis for sickle cell anemia includes penicillin (usually for the first five years) to prevent pneumonia and hydroxyurea to promote development of fetal hemoglobin, which helps to prevent sickling of red blood cells. Blood transfusions are not generally given routinely, although a few clients with high risks of stroke, acute chest syndrome, or ruptured spleen may receive them routinely. Transfusions are more commonly used when anemia worsens or complications such as an enlarged spleen occur. Oxygen is administered when complications such as acute chest syndrome occur.

63. 1: A common response to severe trauma, such as rape, is denial. Clients may at one extreme deny an event has even happened, but more often they exhibit denial by closing down their emotions and remaining calm, insisting that they are "fine" and need no intervention or help. They may try to appear and function as though the event has not happened at all and start "getting on with life," but this is rarely a good solution because they may not adequately deal emotionally with the trauma, resulting in ongoing psychological problems, such as depression, suicidal ideation, flashbacks, and fear.

64. 4: Any time an object has penetrated the eye, it should be left as undisturbed as possible until the client can be examined by an ophthalmologist because removing the object may cause more damage to the eye. Applying a patch or irrigating the eye may disturb the object as well and should be avoided. The client should be positioned on his back with his head elevated, and he may need medication for pain or relaxation while awaiting the consult. A gauze pad may be placed below the eye if tearing is excessive.

65. 3: Because the team leader is ultimately responsible for care that has been delegated to other staff members, the nurse should tell the team leader that she has never changed a tracheostomy tube before and ask for assistance. The team leader should make the decision as to whether he would assist her or assign the task of assisting to another nurse on the team. The nurse should never attempt a procedure for which she is not prepared or knowledgeable.

66. 2, 3, 4, and 5: Foods that are hard or solid and round pose the greatest risk to children one to three years of age because they can easily asphyxiate if the food becomes lodged in the throat. These foods include peanuts, popcorn, round hard candies, and hot dogs. For the same reason, small children should not have access to coins or other small objects that they might put in their mouths and accidentally swallow. Aspiration of foreign objects is the leading cause of accidental death in infants up to one year of age.

67. 3: The most appropriate response to a client who has chosen to receive no treatment is the one that supports the client's choice and provides useful information: "The palliative care and hospice program can help you with comfort measures, such as pain control." The nurse should avoid trying to pressure the client into accepting treatment, and holding out the possibility of a cure for someone with fourth-stage cancer is essentially meaningless. For some clients, having no treatment is the best choice.

68. 1: The response that demonstrates therapeutic communication is "Your pain is not well controlled" because it is restating the implied message that the client is communicating. The nurse should avoid making "should" statements or questioning the client's actions, but she should attempt to explore the issue to determine what intervention is needed. "You poor thing" is not helpful in solving the problem and suggests that the client is a victim rather than an active collaborator in his own care.

69. 4: Unless the adolescent has a cognitive or other physical impairment that interferes with his ability to comprehend, the most appropriate pain assessment tool is the 1-to-10 scale, which is commonly used with adults. The face, legs, activity, cry, consolability (FLACC) scale is appropriate for children from two months to seven years of age. The Wong–Baker FACES tool can be used from ages three on up through adulthood, but it is most appropriate for children before adolescence because of its cartoonish nature.

70. 3, 4, and 6: Dehydration results in the following signs and symptoms:

- Increased urinary specific gravity (>1.028).
- Increased blood urea nitrogen (BUN) and BUN-creatinine ratio.
- Increased hemoglobin and hematocrit.
- Poor skin turgor.
- Dry mucous membranes.
- Weakness and dizziness.
- Tachycardia.
- Fever.

Elderly clients are especially susceptible to dehydration, so their fluid intake should be monitored carefully. Rehydration and replacement of lost electrolytes are critical. Clients may be provided oral rehydration fluids or intravenous (IV) fluids, depending on their condition and ability to tolerate oral fluids.

71. 2: Because standing is the problem that the client is having with showering, the most appropriate suggestion is to use a shower chair. Microwavable disposable cloths for sponge baths are most useful for bedbound clients or for short-term use and are frequently used for hospitalized clients. If the client were unable to actually wash herself because of general weakness, then referral to a home health agency might be appropriate. An occupational therapist may be needed if the client has multiple problems managing activities of daily living (ADLs) in the home environment.

72. 4: Although each person grieves differently, this client's grieving behavior is distorted because she is in a state of prolonged despair that prevents her from working through her grief and finding some resolution. Distorted responses to grief often derive from profound unresolved anger, directed toward oneself and preventing the person from functioning. Clients who had ambivalent feelings toward the deceased may experience prolonged grieving because of guilt and may begin to blame themselves for the person's death.

73. 1: There are four stages of labor:

Stage 1: The period between the onset of labor and full dilation (10 cm). Comprises two phases: latent (cervical effacement and beginning dilation) and active (continued dilation from 4 to 10 cm).
Stage 2: The period from full dilation through the delivery of the infant.
Stage 3: The period after delivery of the infant through delivery of the placenta.
Stage 4: The postpartum period lasting two hours after delivery.

74. 2: A client with a complete spinal cord injury at level C8 is a quadriplegic and should be able to use a manual wheelchair independently on most surfaces but may require adaptive devices for activities of daily living (ADLs). The client should have full extension and flexion of her elbows and wrists and some movement in the fingers and thumbs. She should be able to transfer independently and drive a car with hand controls. The client may need some assistance with ADLs, such as lower body dressing.

75. 3: Lethargy, change in mental status, and asterixis in a client when receiving TPN are indications of hyperammonemia, so the protein concentration of the formula should be decreased, and the client should be evaluated for hepatic insufficiency. Other complications include insertion trauma, thrombus formation, phlebitis, fluid imbalance, hyperglycemia, hypoglycemia, electrolyte imbalance, azotemia, essential fatty acid deficiency, and hyperlipidemia. Formulas that are commercially prepared contain dextrose and protein, but other trace elements, electrolytes, and vitamins are added as well as fat emulsions on an individual basis.

76. 1: Primary graft dysfunction (reperfusion injury) is a major cause of illness and death in lung recipients with symptoms and treatment similar to acute respiratory distress syndrome (ARDS). Indications of primary graft dysfunction include frequent oxygen desaturation, general malaise, increased dyspnea and work associated with the act of breathing, and intolerance to activity. Causes may include increased capillary permeability, interrupted lymphatic drainage, edema, and mismatch in compliance and vascular resistance between the donor and the recipient.

77. 4: Prone position: Blood may pool in the extremities, and pressure on the abdomen may result in a decrease in blood pressure (BP), preload, and cardiac output. Respiratory effort increases, and lung compliance decreases. The head positioned sharply to one side may interfere with cerebral circulation. If the head is turned laterally, the dependent eye must be observed carefully for external compression. Bilateral bolsters or other supports should be used to support the thorax (clavicle to iliac crest) to relieve abdominal compression, which may impede respirations and venous return.

78. 1, 2, 3, and 5: Typical indications that death will occur within a few days include lethargy, disorientation, and increasing dysphagia. Clients are usually unable to take foods or swallow medications. The client appears very weak, gaunt, and pale and is able to take only sips of fluid. Clients usually have decreased urinary output and may be incontinent of concentrated urine. The cardiac rate and respiratory rate both increase, but the strength of cardiac contractions weakens, and the pulse may become irregular.

79. 2: According to federal law, if a client dies in a hospital setting, the staff must ask the family decision maker about organ donation. In some cases, the client will have indicated a preference on an advance directive, but in practice, if family members object, the harvesting of organs is usually not carried out, so it's important that the staff member approaching the family be trained and sensitive to the family members' feelings and concerns. Information about organ donation is often provided to the client and family on admission.

80. 1: The sterile field extends from the waist to the shoulders, and sterile gowns are considered sterile only between these points. Any sterile item that is held out of the line of sight or below the waist is considered contaminated. The sterile field should be placed on a table that is waist high. The drape is considered sterile except for one inch around the perimeter of the drape, so no contents should come in contact with that area. Sterile items should be dropped toward the center of the drape.

81. 830 mL: If a client with deficiency of coagulation factors because of liver disease is to receive 10 mL of fresh frozen plasma per kg of body weight and the client's weight is 183 lb (83 kg), the patient should receive 830 mL of FFP (83 × 10). FFP is usually supplied in 200 mL units, and the required dose is rounded to the nearest unit, so the patient would receive 4 units of FFP. FFP must be ABO/Rh compatible and must be administered within 24 hours of thawing.

82. 1, 3, and 4: The following tests must be performed to diagnose brain death prior to organ donation:

- 2 EEGs taken 12 to 24 hours apart: Total lack of electrical activity
- Testing of brainstem reflexes: pupillary response to light, corneal reflex, vestibular ocular reflex, gag reflex, and motor response to pain
- Apnea test: Usually performed after second testing of brainstem reflexes, but need only be done one time if results are conclusive

If injuries are so severe that they prevent some testing, then other confirmatory testing, such as transcranial Doppler ultrasonography, may be done.

83. 1: If the sister of a client with end-stage kidney disease has stated she will donate a kidney to her brother but actually does not want to do so even though testing shows she is a good match and does not want her brother or family to know she has refused to donate, the best response to the client, who questions this, is: "I don't believe she was a match." While the sister is physically matched, she is not emotionally matched. Because people often feel coerced into donating, the United Network for Organ Sharing (UNOS) has provided guidelines that state that potential donors who do not want to donate should receive a nonspecific statement of unsuitability.

84. 4: Clients may turn down offers of hospice care because they have no clear idea of the benefits and may mistakenly believe that hospice is just there to provide support during death. The nurse should explain the benefits, such as the provision of equipment, supplies, pain medication, and pain control, as well as services by other supportive members of the hospice team, such as home health aides and social workers. The client should be advised that he can contact hospice at any time if he changes his mind.

85. 1, 3, and 4: Post-mortem care includes positioning the limbs in proper alignment, placing dentures in the mouth, and cleansing the body gently (because the tissue is friable after death). The eyelids should be closed, but taping or applying weights is not necessary, and tape may damage tissue. A roll may be placed under the jaw to hold the mouth closed. The body is usually left unclothed. These interventions should be carried out shortly after death because rigor mortis begins within 2 to 4 hours.

86. 4: In the normal electrocardiogram (ECG) complex, the QRS complex represents ventricular depolarization:

- P wave: Start of electrical impulse in the sinus node and spreading through the atria, muscle depolarization
- QRS complex: Ventricular muscle depolarization and atrial repolarization. The width of the complex represents intraventricular conduction time.

- T wave: Ventricular muscle repolarization (resting state) as cells regain negative charge
- U wave: Repolarization of the Purkinje fibers

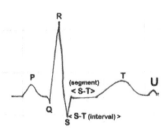

87. 2: If a client has had a ventricular pacemaker implanted, has lethargy, headache, pain in the jaw, breathlessness, and anxiety, and the nurse notes pulsations evident in the neck and the abdomen, the most likely reason is that the client is experiencing mild pacemaker syndrome. This occurs when the timing of atrial and ventricular contractions is not adequately synchronized. With moderate pacemaker syndrome, the client may experience increased dyspnea, orthopnea, dizziness, and confusion. With severe pacemaker syndrome, the client may develop pulmonary edema and heart failure.

88. 4: While a nasogastric tube for decompression is usually placed with the client's head elevated, when gastric lavage is done to remove drugs or poisons, the client is placed in left lateral position with the head lowered 15 degrees because this position causes substances in the stomach to pool and reduces movement of the substances into the duodenum. A large bore tube (36 to 40 Fr) is usually used for gastric lavage and may be placed nasally or orally.

89. 1: If a client's hemoglobin is 6.1 and hematocrit is 18.3 and falling, and he has been advised that he might die but has refused to accept blood transfusions because of religious beliefs, the best response is to provide supportive care as indicated and respect the client's right to refuse treatment. While it is appropriate to tell the client that he can change his mind at any time, pressuring the client or his family is not appropriate.

90. 1: If a client with severe diarrhea, nausea, and vomiting has become increasingly lethargic and weak with tingling in the hands and feet, muscle cramps and tetany, hypotension, and dysrhythmias with ECG abnormalities that include PVCs and flattened T waves, the nurse should suspect hypokalemia. Potassium influences the activity of both skeletal and cardiac muscles. Normal values range from 3.5 to 5.5 mEq/L. Hypokalemia occurs with levels of less than 3.4 mEq/L and critical values of less than 2.5 mEq/L.

91. 3 and 4: The orders that correctly use abbreviations are "Levothyroxine 0.112 mg daily" because the decimal has a leading zero and "acetaminophen 650 mg at HS" because "at" is spelled out rather than using "@," which may be misread as the number 2. The order "MS 10.0 mg SC stat" improperly abbreviates morphine sulfate and has a trailing zero, which can result in the order being misread as "100 mg." "DSS Q.D." uses "Q.D." instead of "daily" or "each day." Abbreviations, such as "TCN" for tetracycline, should be avoided.

92. 4: If the unit supervisor assigns a nurse to three clients for primary care and the nurse discovers that one client is a close neighbor and casual friend, the nurse should immediately inform the supervisor and ask that the client be reassigned. Since the nurse and client have a preexisting social relationship, the client may be uncomfortable with the nurse knowing personal information or providing care but may not be comfortable stating so outright.

93. 1 and 2: HIPAA privacy and security rules protect personal health information about a client, so it is a HIPAA violation to share information about the client with family and friends other than parents of a minor child or a spouse without specific permission to do so. It is a security violation to allow unauthorized access to the EHR, and this includes not only sharing passwords but also allowing others to "shoulder surf" in order to gain information.

94. 2: If the nurse is assigned as team leader for an LVN and 2 CNAs, the tasks that should be assigned to the LVN are the dressing change and insertion of a Foley catheter. Checking routine vital signs, giving enemas, and giving bed baths are all within the scope of practice of CNAs, but facility guidelines may vary. When delegating, the nurse must consider the 5 rights of delegation: right person, right task, right circumstances, right direction, and right supervision.

95. 1, 3, and 6: If a client has been exploring different types of complementary therapies and states, "I don't need to worry about taking herbs because they're natural," the client needs to be aware that many prescription medications are derived from herbs, and herbs may interact with medications and increase or decrease their actions. Additionally, "Homeopathic medicine is better for infections than antibiotics," is not supported by any research and may pose a risk to the client if an infection goes untreated. "I've heard that there is an herbal cure for cancer in Mexico" suggests the client is relying on unsubstantiated claims.

96. 3: If a client has expressed a desire to quit smoking and asks the nurse for advice, the first step that the nurse should suggest is that the client take is to make a quit plan. The client should determine a quit date, preferably within 2 weeks. During that time, the client should inform family and friends, make a list of possible adverse effects (cravings, withdrawal) and plan how a response. The client should review smoking habits (when, where, and how) and make a plan to avoid those situations. On the quit date, the client should throw away all tobacco products.

97. 2, 3, 4, and 5: The American Medical Association has developed guidelines for informed consent. Components include:

- Explanation of diagnosis
- Nature and reason for treatment or procedure
- Risks and benefits
- Alternative options (regardless of cost or insurance coverage)
- Risks and benefits of alternative options
- Risks and benefits of not having a treatment or procedure

Clients should have a good understanding of the procedure itself and the risks and possible complications associated with a procedure. Clients should not in any way be coerced into signing an informed consent form.

98. 2: While there is value in all of these approaches, the best place to begin to gather information about evidence-based practices is to search medical databases, such as Medline Plus, DynaMed Plus, CINAHL, and Cochrane. These resources can provide up-to-date information that is supported by data, critical elements for evidence-based practice. However, the evidence gathered should be carefully assessed for both internal and external validity, including reviewing the numbers of subjects and credentials of the authors.

99. 3: Without being overly technical or overly simplistic ("sound . . . was normal"), the nurse should explain to the daughter that trapped air escaped from the lungs when the client was moved. The nurse should also explain other changes to expect, such as a cooling of the body temperature

(1° to 1.8°C/hour) and discoloring of dependent tissues (liver mortis). In most cases, the client's body is transported to a funeral home prior to the onset of rigor mortis (2 to 4 hours), but the daughter should be advised of this also if the wait time is longer.

100. 1, 2, 3, and 4: If a client is admitted for treatment of a myocardial infarction but insists on leaving against medical advice and the nurse is unable to reach the physician, the nurse should advise the client of health risks of leaving before treatment completed, assess the client's mental status and ability to make decisions, ask the client to sign an AMA form, and arrange for some type of follow-up, such as by phone or return visit. The client should be provided necessary discharge information, such as about treatment provided and the plan of care, as well as contact information for the physician or other healthcare provider.

101. 2: If a physician has telephoned a number of orders for a client who has developed a fever and chills, the nurse should write the orders in their entirety and then read back and confirm that the orders are correct. However, if an order is not clear, then the nurse should clarify that order when it is given. The nurse may repeat the individual orders while writing them, but should not routinely stop with each order to confirm as this interrupts the physician's flow of thought and may be distracting.

102. 1: If an 11-year-old child with autism spectrum disorder is hospitalized but is frequently extremely agitated, refusing to take medications and screaming and hitting his head against the bed headboard, especially when the parents are not present, the nurse should ask the parents for advice about managing the child's behavior because comfort measures may be very individual with autism. If possible, at least one parent should remain with the child at all times.

103. 1: If an elderly client hospitalized for a stroke from a long-term care facility has a large diamond ring that is very loose and has fallen off of the client's finger twice, the nurse should remove the ring and secure it according to hospital policy. Most facilities have a secure safe or other area to store valuables until other arrangements can be made. The ring should not be sent home with a family member or caregiver unless this person has power of attorney, is the parent of a client who is a minor, or is a spouse.

104. 4: If a nurse has removed running sutures with 8 stitches (including the knotted stitch at the top and bottom), when the suture removal is complete, the nurse should have removed eight individual pieces of suture. Although the running suture comprises one long piece of suture material, each stitch in the line must be removed individually because suture material that is on the outside of the skin cannot be pulled through the tissue as it may be contaminated with bacteria.

105. 3: If a patient who underwent a fiberoptic bronchoscopy for a right lung biopsy develops dyspnea, ipsilateral pain, increased pulse rate, hypotension, and coughing during the recovery period, the most likely reason is pneumothorax or bleeding. The nurse should immediately assess the client's lungs to determine if the breath sounds are diminished and notify the physician of the changes in condition. The physician will likely order a chest x-ray and a hemoglobin and hematocrit.

106. 2: If monitoring a client's control of diabetes, the most reliable source of information is the client's HbA1c, which indicates the average level of glucose over a 3-month period. The serum glucose level can change from day to day depending on carbohydrate intake and various other factors, so it is less reliable. While the client's diet and exercise log and report can provide valuable information, clients are not always accurate or honest with reports.

107. 3: If a client with bipolar disorder is exhibiting disturbed thought processes as evidenced by delusional thinking, the nurse should avoid arguing or challenging the client, but should indicate acceptance and reasonable doubt: "I understand you believe this, but I don't see evidence that this is true." The nurse should try to refocus the client's thoughts to reality by talking about real events and people rather than allowing the client to continue to focus on the delusion.

108. 1: When doing nasotracheal suctioning, the catheter should be inserted only during inhalation because during this phase of respiration the epiglottis is open. However, suction should not be applied during insertion. During suctioning, a normal reaction is for the client to cough, but if the client begins to gag or becomes nauseated, the catheter may be in the esophagus. Tracheal suctioning should be completed before pharyngeal because the pharynx contains more bacteria than the trachea.

109. 3: When changing a colostomy appliance, the skin about the stoma should be cleansed with warm tap water. Alcohol may be irritating to the tissue, and soap or baby wipes may leave residue on the tissue that interferes with adhesion. If any soap is used, it should be mild and without oils or perfume and should be rinsed off thoroughly with warm water. If skin paste is present, it should be removed before wetting the skin.

110. 4: While there are some similarities in all levels of alcohol withdrawal, the timeframe (1 week after the last drink) suggests that this is the onset of delirium tremens, which usually manifests on day 3 to day 10 after the last drink and can be life-threatening. DTs are characterized by severe confusion, agitation, hallucinations, hypertension, tachycardia, and fever. Various supportive therapies are used in the treatment of DTs, but the most commonly used drug therapy is benzodiazepines.

111. 37.5 milligrams: If a 7-month-old infant with community-acquired pneumonia (*H. influenzae*) has received a loading dose of azithromycin oral suspension at dosage of 10 mg/kg of body weight (75 mg) on day one in the emergency department and is now to receive 5 mg/kg/day on days 2 to 5, the first step is to change the child's weight from pounds to kilograms: 16.5/2.2 = 7.5. Then, the total weight in kilograms is multiplied by the milligrams per kilogram: 5 × 7.5 = 37.5 milligrams.

112. 2: If a nurse examining the blisters of a client in the active phase of herpes zoster (shingles) has direct contact with bare hands to the fluid in some of the blisters, the nurse is at risk of developing varicella zoster virus (chickenpox) if not previously vaccinated. Shingles results from reactivation of the varicella zoster virus, so in order to develop shingles, the individual must first be infected with chickenpox. Once the blisters of shingles have crusted over, the client is no longer contagious.

113. 4: If a mother is concerned that her neonate is having periods of apnea, the nurse should reassure her that slight pauses in breathing, referred to as periodic breathing, are normal in the neonate. Usually the pause is only 2 or 3 seconds, but it may be longer in some cases. However, if the periods persist for greater than 15 to 20 seconds or increase in frequency, the mother should notify the physician, especially if the episodes are accompanied by other changes, such as pallor, cyanosis, bradycardia, or hypotonia.

114. 3: If a client who has never received a measles vaccination was exposed to a child with measles 14 days earlier, the client is at risk for another 7 days as the incubation period ranges from 7 to 21 days (average onset is at 14 days). Additionally, if the client is infected, she can pass the disease to others from 4 days prior to onset of rash to 4 days after. Measles is an airborne disease, and is spread by body fluids. If an infected person coughs and spreads the virus, the virus can remain airborne for an hour.

115. 1, 4, and 5: If a client falls to the floor with a seizure, the nurse should avoid restraining the client or trying to insert a padded tongue blade between the teeth because this may increase injuries but should try to position the client on one side with the head flexed slightly forward and should support the head with cushioning of some sort to prevent head injury. Constrictive clothing should be loosened. As much as possible, the client should be provided privacy.

116. 4: If a client is experiencing hypothermia, treatment depends on the core body temperature. For temperatures ranging from less than 28°C to 32.2°C, active internal rewarming procedures are carried out. These include cardiopulmonary bypass, warm IV fluid administration, and warm peritoneal lavage. However, for temperatures ranging from 32.2°C to 35°C, passive or active external rewarming procedures are used. These include over-the-bed heaters and forced air warm blankets. Patients with hypothermia have reduced sensation, so they must be carefully monitored to prevent burns.

117. 2, 3, and 5: If the nurse is examining a client's incision following a radical nephrectomy, signs or symptoms that may be indicative of infection include tissue about the incision being moderately edematous and increasingly erythematous, the dressing that has covered the wound having a foul odor, and evidence of purulent discharge. Slight serosanguineous discharge is common and usually no cause for concern. Pain in the incisional area in the postoperative period is very common and usually does not indicate infection unless there is a change in the character of the pain and other signs or symptoms are present.

118. 3: The dressing type that is most appropriate for a stage II pressure ulcer with moderate amounts of exudate is the hydrocolloid dressing, which contains gelling agents, which help to absorb exudate. NS and gauze (wet-to-dry) dressings are no longer recommended because they disturb granulating tissue. Transparent film is not appropriate for exudative wounds because it has no absorptive properties. Hydrogel dressings are designed to hydrate dry wounds and are not used for wounds with exudate.

119. 1, 2, 3, and 5: Peritoneal dialysis is usually done with about 2 L of dialysate, so this means that at all times, the client retains about 2 L of fluid, which may result in slight abdominal distention. Most clients do 4 to 5 exchanges in a 24-hour period with a longer period of retention during the night. Each exchange usually takes 30 to 40 minutes. Because the fluid flows into the peritoneal cavity, the client is at risk of peritonitis, so the client must use sterile procedures.

120. 3 and 4: Negative pressure wound therapy (NPWT) requires skilled nursing both for removal and application, so these tasks cannot be delegated to UAP nor can wound assessment. However, the nurse should provide instructions to UAP so that they are aware that they should report any changes in the client's comfort level or any elevation of temperature, which could indicate infection. Also, the UAP must monitor the tubing to prevent displacement when turning the client.

Practice Test #3

1. A client with end-stage heart failure is bedridden, and the skin in the coccygeal area is red and tender despite frequent turning because the client is occasionally incontinent of urine. The client weighs 180 pounds. Which type of pressure-relieving surface should the nurse most recommend at this time?

    1. foam overlay
    2. sheepskin
    3. alternating pressure overlay
    4. low air loss bed

2. A client is to receive 120 mL of normal saline per hour intravenously. The drop factor is 15 drops per mL. What drip rate should the nurse set? *Record your answer using a whole number.*

3. A client has weakness of both lower extremities, more pronounced on the right, and uses crutches to ambulate. Which of the following gaits requires the most upper body strength and balance?

    1. 4-point
    2. 3-point
    3. 2-point
    4. swing-through

4. A client has just had a long leg cast applied to his left leg and is in bed. The cast is still damp, and the client is cold. Which of the following actions by the nurse are appropriate? Select all that apply.

    1. cover the client, including the cast, with a warm blanket
    2. cover the client with a warm blanket, leaving the cast exposed to the air
    3. place a high-powered electric fan to blow directly on the cast
    4. turn and reposition the client every 2 to 3 hours
    5. place a fan in the room but directed away from the client

5. The nurse is administering an intermittent tube feeding to a client per an NG tube. The nurse has checked placement of the tube, checked for gastric residual, and aspirated 150 mL of gastric contents. Which of the following next actions is most appropriate?

    1. hold feeding and notify MD of gastric residual
    2. proceed with tube feeding
    3. return the aspirated gastric contents to the stomach and flush the tubing with 30 mL water
    4. return 100 mL of aspirated gastric contents to the stomach followed by the tube feeding

6. The physician has ordered that a client with diabetes insipidus receive 50 micrograms of desmopressin acetate by oral tabs twice daily. The tablets are labeled 0.2 mg per tablet. How many tablets will the nurse administer for each dose? *Record your answer using a decimal number.*

7. Following surgical removal of an ovarian cyst, a client has not urinated in 4 hours and feels the urge to urinate but is unable to initiate urine flow. Which of the following should the nurse do initially to promote urination? Select all that apply.

1. pour warm water over the client's perineum while she is on the toilet
2. ask the client to blow bubbles through a straw into a glass of water while trying to urinate
3. turn on running water while the client tries to urinate
4. tell the client to "just relax"
5. catheterize the client

8. An adult client has instilled drops into the ear to soften cerumen, and the nurse is to irrigate the ear to remove the cerumen. Which of the following statements are correct about ear irrigations? Select all that apply.

1. 50 mL of irrigant should be instilled at one time
2. the tip of the syringe should be used to occlude the ear canal
3. the pinna should be pulled up and back
4. allow fluid to drain out during the procedure
5. position client in sitting or lying position
6. ask client to turn the head away from the affected ear

9. A client receiving chemotherapy for breast cancer (stage 2) tells the nurse that she is considering complementary therapy to relieve her almost constant nausea and asks the nurse for advice. Which of the following complementary therapies is most likely to be safe and effective?

1. acupuncture
2. therapeutic touch
3. magnetic therapy
4. herbal therapies

10. The nurse asks a Hispanic immigrant to evaluate his pain on a scale of one to ten, and the client states his pain is at level one. However, the client looks distressed and is bent over and rubbing his stomach. Which of the following approaches by the nurse is most indicated?

1. use a different type of questioning to ascertain pain level
2. accept the client's word about pain
3. tell the client he appears to be minimizing his discomfort
4. ask the client if he is afraid to admit to pain

11. A client is in cervical traction for a herniated cervical disc. The client complains of increasing pain in the jaw and both ears. Which of the following interventions is most indicated?

1. provide increased analgesia
2. adjust weights
3. correct head position
4. correct body position

12. The nurse calls a physician to report a client's sudden increase in temperature and receives a telephone order for an antibiotic. Which of the following is the correct procedure for the nurse?

1. write the telephone order, order from the pharmacy, and administer the medication
2. write the telephone order, read it back, and ask for verbal verification before ordering the drug from the pharmacy and administering the medication
3. write the order, repeating it back, and then order the drug from the pharmacy and administer the medication
4. write the order and check with a supervisor before ordering the drug from the pharmacy and administering the medication

13. The nurse believes he observes another nurse taking an opioid medication intended for a client. Which of the following initial actions is the most appropriate?

1. confront the nurse taking the client's medication
2. notify a supervisor about the observation
3. notify the client's physician
4. carry out a personal investigation

14. The nurse is working in the emergency department. Which of the following injuries must be reported to the police or appropriate authorities?

1. a woman has multiple facial injuries and defensive wounds on the hands and arms but insists she fell
2. a 6-year-old child has severe head and face injuries and multiple broken ribs. X-rays indicate numerous old orthopedic injuries, and the mother states the child fell off a swing
3. a client has a large open cut on his torso and claims he was injured when a large light fixture fell on him
4. an 18-year-old girl who was severely intoxicated from drinking fell and broke her arm

15. A hospitalized client calls the nurse into the room and reports that another nurse has been rude to her. Which of the following initial responses by the nurse is most appropriate?

1. "I'm sure the nurse didn't mean to be rude."
2. "The nurse was probably just very busy."
3. "I'm sorry! There's no excuse for a nurse being rude."
4. "I'm so sorry you felt that way. Can you tell me what happened?"

16. The nurse is documenting the interview with a client with asthma and diabetes. Which of the following documentations is correct? Select all that apply.

1. "Client appears SOB and anxious."
2. "Client took nebulizer treatment with .25 mg budesonide inhalation suspension prior to visit."
3. "Client needs new prescription for 0.5% albuterol inhalation solution."
4. "Client checks blood sugar Q.O.D."
5. "Client exhibits dyspnea and tachypnea (26/min)."

17. A mother's amniotic fluid is meconium stained. Which of the following complications does the nurse anticipate the neonate may develop?

1. anemia
2. respiratory distress
3. growth retardation
4. cognitive impairment

18. Which of the following ensures minimal proper identification prior to administering medication?

1. nurse recognizes client
2. nurse asks client's name and checks hospital ID bracelet
3. nurse reads client's name on intake and output record at the foot of the client's bed
4. nurse asks client's name

19. A wheelchair-bound client is to be discharged from a rehabilitation facility to the home environment. He still needs minimal assistance for transfers because he is unable to stand and is concerned about transferring from the wheelchair to the toilet and back. Which of the following assistive devices is most indicated to facilitate safe transfer?

1. gait/transfer belt
2. full-body sling lift
3. caregiver assistance only
4. sliding board

20. A nurse must retrieve supplies on the top shelf of a supply room but cannot reach the shelf, which is about a foot above the nurse's reach. Which of the following is an acceptable work practice?

1. stand on a footstool
2. use a ladder
3. climb onto a chair
4. step onto the second shelf of the cabinet

21. The nurse receives a delivery of a container with this marking (see diagram).

What is the meaning of this international symbol?

1. poison
2. medical equipment
3. biohazard
4. radioactive

22. A client with diabetes mellitus type 2 is being discharged, and the nurse is instructing the client about safe disposal of syringes and needles at home. Which of the following information should the nurse provide when educating the client? Select all that apply.

1. "Place needles and syringes in a sharps disposal container immediately after use."
2. "Keep the container in a safe place out of reach of children and pets."
3. "Dispose of the sharps container in the regular trash can."
4. "Dispose of the sharps container in accordance with community guidelines."
5. "Dispose of the sharps container when it is three-quarters full."
6. "Needles can be flushed down the toilet."

23. The hospital receives news that a train has crashed one-half mile away and that a cloud of nonlethal hazardous material has blanketed the area. Which of the following emergency responses does the nurse anticipate?

1. evacuation
2. shelter in place
3. relocation of staff and clients to interior of building
4. partial evacuation—children and critically ill only

24. The nurse is caring for a client with severe diarrhea and fecal incontinence from a *Clostridium difficile* infection. Which of the following infection control precautions should the nurse expect to implement? Select all that apply.

1. use ≥N95 respirators while caring for client
2. use personal protective equipment (gown and gloves) for all contacts with the client
3. maintain client in a private room or >3 feet away from other patients
4. wash hands with soap and water rather than alcohol antiseptics
5. wear masks for all contacts with the client
6. avoid sharing electronic thermometers used by the client with other clients

25. A 15-month-old child who weighs 10 kg is being treated with amoxicillin oral suspension at the rate of 25 mg/kg/day in two divided doses 12 hours apart. How many milligrams should the child receive at each dose? *Record your answer using a whole number only.*

26. A hospital must be evacuated because of flooding in the area. The nurse is working in the neonatal nursery and has been advised to utilize the Safe Babies® apron to transfer infants. How many infants does the nurse anticipate can be moved in one trip in the apron pockets?

1. two
2. four
3. six
4. eight

27. The nurse is about to conduct a bedside electrocardiogram of a client experiencing chest pain, but she notes that the electrical cord is frayed near the plug. Which of the following actions is most indicated?

1. conduct the ECG but then label the ECG machine as "Out of Order"
2. place tape about the frayed cord and conduct the ECG
3. call for repair of the ECG machine
4. immediately obtain a second ECG machine and conduct the ECG

28. The nurse is working as a team leader and discussing assignments with team members. Which of the following statements to the group by a team member is a HIPAA violation of privacy?

    1. "Mrs. Brown says she has no support system when she goes home."
    2. "Mrs. Brown says she has been having an affair with her husband's brother!"
    3. "Mrs. Brown says she dislikes her therapist, so she refuses to cooperate."
    4. "Mrs. Brown seems angry all of the time and yells at her family when they visit."

29. The nurse must give a client a nebulizer treatment every 4 hours. When is the most appropriate time to document the treatments in the electronic health record?

    1. at the beginning of the nurse's shift
    2. immediately after each treatment
    3. within 2 hours of each treatment
    4. at the end of the nurse's shift

30. A homeless client has been treated in the emergency department for a small cut received in a fight with another homeless person and is about to be discharged after suturing. Which of the following information would be most helpful for the client in addition to information about wound care and a follow-up appointment?

    1. telephone number for Adult Protective Services
    2. telephone number of the police department
    3. list of shelters and community agencies
    4. list of 12-step organizations

31. A nurse is concerned that current procedures for wound care are not adequate and would like to propose changes. When pursuing process improvement, where should the nurse begin?

    1. survey literature regarding wound care
    2. conduct interviews of physicians
    3. dispense staff questionnaires
    4. ask permission of the director of nursing

32. A client is no longer responding to curative treatments. What is the best approach to initiating a discussion about the referral to palliative and hospice care?

    1. "Further treatment is not going to help you."
    2. "Would you like to transfer to palliative and hospice care?"
    3. "Have you thought about stopping all treatments?"
    4. "What do you understand about your options for care?"

33. A client has undergone gastric bypass surgery but is experiencing severe dumping syndrome after eating. Which of the following should the nurse advise the client to avoid? Select all that apply.

    1. concentrated sugars
    2. fluids with meals
    3. whole milk and yogurt
    4. reclining after eating
    5. large meals

34. A client tells the nurse that he wants to designate his son to make only his healthcare decisions in the event that he is not able to do so, but he is unsure what document he needs to complete. Which of the following should the nurse advise?

1. Living Will
2. Advance Directive
3. Power of Attorney
4. Durable Power of Attorney for Healthcare

35. The nurse is preparing a mother and neonate for discharge. When educating the parents about infant car seats, which of the following information should the nurse include? Select all that apply.

1. "Rear-facing car seats are safer than forward-facing car seats."
2. "Carefully examine a car seat involved in an accident before using again."
3. "The safest positioning of a car seat is in the middle of the back seat."
4. "The neonate's neck should be straight, avoiding the chin-on-chest position."
5. "The harness should be secured until only 3 or 4 fingers slide easily underneath."

36. A parent tells the nurse that her children, 5 and 10 years old, have been complaining of anal itching and have been sleeping poorly and complaining of occasional abdominal pain and nausea. What diagnostic test does the nurse anticipate?

1. complete blood count
2. tape test
3. abdominal x-ray
4. carbon urea breath test

37. A gang member who killed two children in a shooting is hospitalized under police guard and recovering from a gunshot wound. Which of the following violates the ANA Code of Ethics for Nurses?

1. a nurse provides basic care but refuses to talk to the client
2. a nurse asks to be assigned to a different client
3. a nurse asks to take vacation time to avoid caring for the client
4. a nurse tells the team leader that he feels conflicted about caring for the client

38. A patient has undergone an elective abortion, and according to hospital rules, a nurse who is morally opposed to abortions was excused from caring for the patient. However, the patient's assigned nurse is off of the floor, and as the nurse passes by the patient's room, the patient calls out, "Help, I think I'm bleeding!" Which of the following actions by the nurse is correct?

1. tell the patient the nurse will find another nurse to examine her
2. call the nurse assigned to the patient and ask the nurse to return to examine the patient
3. examine the patient for bleeding
4. contact a supervisor

39. A new mother transferring from the delivery room to her room on the unit asks the nurse if her infant will need any immunizations before they are discharged. Which of the following immunizations should the nurse advise the mother the child will require within 12 hours of birth?

    1. polio
    2. heptavalent pneumococcal conjugate
    3. hepatitis B
    4. rotavirus

40. Which of the following are examples of positive reinforcement for a client with anorexia? Select all that apply.

    1. the nurse tells the client, "If you don't stay with the program, you won't make progress"
    2. the client is granted an additional hour of Internet use after eating all her dinner
    3. the nurse tells the client, "You are making good progress"
    4. the client gains one-half pound
    5. the client loses privileges for losing one-half pound

41. The nurse must give an intramuscular injection to an adult. What length of needle is most appropriate?

    1. 0.5 inch
    2. 0.625 inch
    3. 1 inch
    4. 1.5 inches

42. Which of the following pulmonary changes are associated with aging? Select all that apply.

    1. decreased pulmonary elasticity
    2. increased alveolar surface area
    3. increased chest-wall rigidity
    4. increased forced vital capacity
    5. decreased laryngeal reflexes

43. A 52-year-old client tells the nurse that her yearly Pap smears have always been negative, and she asks if she needs continue to have a Pap smear yearly. Which of the following is the best recommendation?

    1. "You should continue with yearly Pap smears."
    2. "You should have Pap smears every two to three years."
    3. "You should have Pap smears every five years."
    4. "You no longer need to have Pap smears."

44. A 66-year-old monogamous male with low risk factors states that he has not had a physical examination or any medical care for 15 years and asks the nurse if he needs immunizations. Which of the following immunizations should the nurse recommend? Select all that apply.

1. influenza vaccination.
2. pneumococcal vaccination.
3. tetanus-diphtheria booster.
4. herpes zoster (shingles) vaccination.
5. human papillomavirus (HPV) vaccination.
6. mumps, measles, rubella (MMR) vaccination.

45. Which of the following types of cancer is the most common cause of death from cancer for females between the ages of 15 and 34?

1. breast
2. lung
3. cervical
4. ovarian

46. To facilitate the client's right of autonomy, which of the following assessments by the nurse is the most important?

1. the client's cognitive ability
2. legal obligations
3. the physician's wishes
4. the client's physical ability

47. The nurse should advise a client who plans to get pregnant to take which of the following vitamins or minerals to prevent neural tube defects?

1. vitamin D
2. vitamin B_9 (folic acid)
3. vitamin C
4. iron

48. A pregnant client is at term and in the first stages of labor, and the nurse is monitoring the fetal heart rate. Which of the following is the normal fetal heart rate at term?

1. 60 to 90 beats per minute (bpm)
2. 90 to 100 (bpm)
3. 120 to 160 (bpm)
4. 160 to 200 (bpm)

49. A pregnant client nearing term is experiencing Braxton Hicks contractions (false labor). Which of the following indications are characteristic of Braxton Hicks contractions? Select all that apply.

1. associated with dilation of the cervix
2. associated with no dilation of the cervix
3. discomfort is felt over the uterine fundus, radiating to the lower abdomen and back
4. contractions may become rhythmic
5. contractions tend to become longer in duration and at closer intervals of time
6. contractions may resolve with ambulation or pain medication

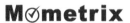

50. Which of the following is the primary purpose in the nurse administering the Apgar (appearance, pulse, grimace, activity, respiration) test to a neonate?

    1. determine the infant's biophysical profile
    2. determine if the infant needs emergency medical care
    3. determine if the infant has congenital defects
    4. determine if the infant is preterm, full term, or post-term

51. A pregnant client tells the nurse that she is Rh– and her husband is Rh+, but she believes she does not need to receive RhoGAM® with a first pregnancy. Which of the following is the best response?

    1. "You are right, but you will need the treatment during a second pregnancy."
    2. "You need treatment during your first pregnancy to prevent Rh incompatibility reactions during a second pregnancy."
    3. "You are wrong. You need the treatment with your first pregnancy."
    4. "You should ask the doctor about that."

52. The nurse is discussing the use of condoms with a 19-year-old male. Which of the following information should the nurse include about latex condom use? Select all that apply.

    1. latex condoms should be used with nonoxynol-9
    2. latex condoms should be used for every act of oral, vaginal, and anal sex
    3. oil-based lubricants may be used with latex condoms
    4. condoms should be removed immediately after ejaculation before the penis becomes flaccid
    5. a condom may be left in place and used for two acts of sex if the acts occur within 30 minutes of each other
    6. condoms provide 100% protection against pregnancy, *human immunodeficiency virus* (HIV), and sexually transmitted diseases (STDs)

53. Which of the following are examples of personal protective equipment (PPE)? Select all that apply.

    1. back belt
    2. goggles
    3. personal radiation dosimeter
    4. respirator
    5. gloves

54. A client tells the nurse that she was recently bitten on the hand by a bat that was inside her house, but the wound has healed. Based on this information, what should the nurse advise the client?

    1. no further treatment is necessary
    2. the client must see a physician immediately because the client is at risk for rabies
    3. the client should see a physician because a latent bacterial infection may occur
    4. the client should see the physician if she develops any symptoms

55. A 26-year-old female who has been hospitalized because of injuries sustained during a robbery is preparing for discharge and tells the nurse that she works as a prostitute and was beaten by a customer. Which of the following is the best response?

1. "Prostitution is illegal! Don't you want to do something else with your life?"
2. "You should stop before you get killed."
3. "I'm sorry. That must be very difficult."
4. "Would you like information about community programs available to help you be safer?"

56. When giving an intramuscular injection, which site should the nurse avoid in obese adults?

1. ventrogluteal
2. deltoid
3. dorsogluteal
4. vastus lateralis

57. A client receiving packed red blood cells complains of itching and is developing hives and local erythema around the IV insertion site.

I. notify the physician
II. stop the transfusion
III. notify the blood bank
IV. administer medications as ordered

Place the actions (in Roman numerals) in the correct order from the first to the last.

1. (First)
2. (Second)
3. (Third)
4. (Fourth)

58. A client is to receive 125 mg of meperidine stat. A vial of meperidine contains 50 mg/mL. How many milliliters are required to provide a dosage of 125 mg? *Record your answer using one decimal place.*

59. The nurse has inserted a Foley catheter into a male client who is bedridden. Which of the following is the best position in which to secure the catheter?

1. the penis is positioned down with the Foley catheter taped to the front of the inner thigh, and then the tubing is looped to allow for turning and it is taped to the edge of the bed
2. the penis is positioned up with the Foley catheter taped to the right or left lower abdomen, and then the tubing is looped to allow for turning and it is taped to the edge of the bed
3. the penis is left unpositioned with the catheter curved over one leg, and the tubing is looped and secured only to the edge of the bed
4. the penis is positioned downward with the catheter secured to the posterior thigh, and the tubing is looped and secured to the edge of the bed

60. The nurse is educating a 23-year-old client about oral contraceptives. Which of the following should the nurse counsel the client to avoid?

1. drinking alcohol
2. smoking
3. eating a high-fat diet
4. doing aerobic exercises

61. The nurse is assisting a client to sit on the side of her bed with the bed in the low position.

> I. support the client until she is stable
>
> II. pivot the client by moving her legs over the side of the bed and elevating her trunk
>
> III. place the client's upper arm across her chest and roll her to a side-lying position toward the nurse by pulling and supporting her shoulders and hips
>
> IV. place one arm under the client's shoulders, supporting her head and neck, and place the other arm over her thighs
>
> V. raise the head of the bed to 30° with the client in the supine position

Place the steps (in Roman numerals) in the correct order from first to last.

> 1. (First)
> 2. (Second)
> 3. (Third)
> 4. (Fourth)
> 5. (Fifth)

62. The client is caring for a client who is awaiting open reduction and internal fixation (ORIF) of a hip fracture and is temporarily immobilized with Buck's traction. The nurse notes that the knot of the rope is lodged against the pulley. What is the primary concern with this finding?

> 1. there is no concern because this is the correct placement of the knot
> 2. this may change body alignment
> 3. this may interfere with the line of pull
> 4. this may change the direction of pull

63. The nurse must empty a Hemovac® on a postoperative client.

> I. open the plug on the port
>
> II. hold the Hemovac over the container and tilt the port toward the container so that fluid drains into the container
>
> III. place the plug into the port
>
> IV. cleanse the plug and the port with an alcohol wipe in the dominant hand while compressing and holding the top and bottom of the Hemovac together with the other hand
>
> V. wash hands and apply gloves

Place the steps (in Roman numerals) to emptying the Hemovac in the correct order from first to last.

> 1. (First)
> 2. (Second)
> 3. (Third)
> 4. (Fourth)
> 5. (Fifth)

64. The nurse must administer 5 ml of acetaminophen solution through the nasogastric (NG) tube of a client, but the NG tube is attached to suction. How long (in minutes) should the nurse discontinue the suction after administering the medication? **Record your answer using a whole number.**

65. The nurse has to apply a warm moist compress to an abscessed area on the back of a client's neck. What is the temperature range for a warm compress?

1. 37 to 41° C/98 to 106° F.
2. 34 to 37° C/93 to 98° F.
3. 26 to 34° C/80 to 93° F.
4. 18 to 26° C/65 to 80° F.

66. What physiological responses should the nurse expect when applying cold compresses to tissue? Select all that apply.

1. local anesthesia
2. increased permeability of the capillaries
3. increased viscosity of the blood
4. increased tissue metabolism
5. decrease in muscle tension
6. vasoconstriction

67. The nurse must collect a urine sample for a routine urinalysis from a client who has had an indwelling self-sealing rubber Foley catheter for three days. After initially clamping the catheter tubing for 20 minutes, which of the following is the correct procedure?

1. the nurse collects a urine sample by opening the tube and draining urine from the collection bag
2. the nurse uses a 20-mL syringe with a 1-inch 21-gauge needle to withdraw urine from the catheter just above where it connects to the drainage tube
3. the nurse disconnects the Foley catheter from the drainage tube and allows urine to drip from the catheter into a sterile urine specimen container
4. the nurse uses a 3-mL syringe with a 1-inch 21-gauge needle to withdraw urine from the catheter near the urinary meatus

68. The nurse is educating the parents of a severely allergic child about methods of controlling dust mites. Which of the following actions should the nurse advise the parents are essential? Select all that apply.

1. keep the house clean and free of obvious dust and clutter
2. encase the child's mattress and box spring in allergen-proof covers
3. remove all carpets from the house
4. replace all upholstered furniture with leather or vinyl furniture
5. wash bed linens, pillows, clothing, and stuffed toys in hot water once a week
6. maintain humidity below 50%

69. A 76-year-old female tells the nurse that she and her husband want to continue to engage in sexual activity, but both have osteoarthritis and limited mobility. Which position should the nurse recommend that will be putting the least strain on both partners?

1. "missionary" position (male on top)
2. female on top
3. "spooning" position with male behind female, side lying
4. rear vaginal entry with female prone and male on top

70. A client with moderately advanced Alzheimer's disease believes that her deceased husband is living with her and frequently "talks" to him about the happy things they do together. Which is the best nursing response?

1. tell the client that her husband has died
2. try to distract the client when she discusses her husband
3. ask the physician for medication to help control the client's hallucinations and delusions
4. allow the client to believe that her husband is alive

71. A client is recovering from placement of an implantable cardioverter-defibrillator (ICD) and suddenly exhibits hypotension with narrowing pulse pressure, pulsus paradoxus, distant heart sounds, restlessness, bulging neck veins, and increasing cyanosis. Which of the following is the most likely cause of these signs and symptoms?

1. perforation of the ventricle with cardiac tamponade
2. incorrect positioning of the leads
3. myocardial infarction
4. heart failure

72. Following a myocardial infarction, enzymes and proteins are released into the blood. In what order would the nurse expect to see the enzyme and protein levels rise, peak, and return to normal? Place the following enzymes/proteins (in Roman numerals) in the correct order in the chart below.

I. troponin T.
II. creatine kinase (CK)-MB
III. troponin I
IV. myoglobin

Enzyme/Protein	Rise	Peak	Return to normal
(1)	2 hours	4 hours	24 hours
(2)	4–8 hours	20 hours	≤72
(3)	3–6 hours	14–20 hours	5 to 7 days
(4)	3–6 hours	12–24 hours	10 to 15 days

73. The nurse is providing education about Raynaud's disease to a 35-year-old female client. Which of the following information should the nurse include? Select all that apply.

1. stop smoking (make a referral to a smoking cessation program)
2. wear mittens and gloves when outside during cold weather
3. handle cold items from the refrigerator or freezer for brief periods only
4. avoid calcium channel blockers
5. avoid vasodilators
6. avoid birth control pills

74. The nurse is assessing a client's cardiac monitoring and notes the following electrocardiogram (ECG) recording:

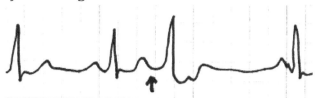

How would the nurse classify this cardiac abnormality?

1. atrial flutter
2. premature junctional contraction
3. ventricular tachycardia
4. premature ventricular contraction

75. A client's blood pressure is 156/92. What is the pulse pressure in mm Hg? **Record your answer using a whole number.**

76. A client with a brain tumor has exhibited changes in mood and personality and has developed weakness on her right side. Based on these symptoms, the nurse suspects the tumor is located in which part of the brain?

1. occipital lobe
2. frontal lobe
3. temporal lobe
4. cerebellum

77. A client with a head injury is being admitted into the intensive care unit with a score on the Glasgow Coma Scale of 6. Based on this score, what condition does the nurse anticipate?

1. mild head injury
2. severe head injury
3. coma
4. moderate head injury

78. The nurse is caring for four clients, all of whom need attention:

I. six-hour postoperative client is asking for pain medication for pain of 8 on a scale of 1 to 10
II. two-day postoperative client needs a routine dressing change
III. five-day postoperative client needs intermittent tube feeding
IV. three-day postoperative client needs assessment for sudden elevated temperature

Prioritize the clients (in Roman numerals) according to the order in which the nurse should attend to them.

1. (First) _____
2. (Second) _____
3. (Third) _____
4. (Fourth) _____

79. Nurse A notes that nurse B on the unit smells of alcohol and is slightly slurring her words. What is the best course of action for nurse A?

1. tell nurse B that she needs to go home because she appears to be inebriated
2. immediately notify a supervisor
3. observe nurse B to ensure that she is providing safe care
4. assist nurse B in caring for her clients until she is less impaired

80. A client has developed signs of tardive dyskinesia with repetitive behavior, including lip smacking and tongue protrusion with choreiform movements of the trunk and extremities. Which of the following medications is most likely the cause of these symptoms?

1. donepezil HCl (Aricept®)
2. fluoxetine HCl (Prozac®)
3. celecoxib (Celebrex®)
4. haloperidol (Haldol®)

81. A client with 2+ peripheral edema and increasing complaints of lethargy has the following laboratory results:

Test	Result
BUN	172 mg/dL
Serum creatinine	16.4 mg/dL
Glucose	98 mg/dL

Which further testing does the nurse expect based on these findings?

1. testing for diabetes
2. testing for liver disease
3. testing results are inconclusive
4. testing for kidney disease

82. If the nurse is to give a client two oral medications (capsules) per the enteral feeding tube, which of the following is the correct procedure?

1. open the capsules directly into the feeding formula and instill
2. open the capsules together and dilute with water before instilling
3. open the capsules separately and dilute each with water before instilling
4. oral medications cannot be given per the enteral feeding tube

83. Which of the following are age-related changes that typically occur in the respiratory system? Select all that apply.

1. blunting of cough/laryngeal reflexes
2. alveoli fewer in number
3. decreased ciliary action
4. alveoli smaller in size
5. increased elasticity of lung tissue
6. increased rigidity of thoracic muscles

84. When assessing a client's health history regarding intake of alcohol, which of the following would qualify the person as an "at-risk" drinker?

1. a male client goes out with friends 1 or 2 times a week and has 4 to 6 drinks
2. a female client rarely drinks but "got drunk" at a college party 4 years earlier
3. a male client typically has 2 glasses of wine each day
4. a female client typically has 5 to 6 beers per week

96

85. **Two years after the death of her spouse, a client remains preoccupied with memories of her deceased husband, neglecting family and friends. Which of the following types of grief response is the client experiencing?**

1. inhibited
2. distorted
3. prolonged
4. normal

86. **A client with a long history of alcohol abuse has been prescribed disulfiram so that he will stop drinking. When educating the client about the acetaldehyde syndrome, which of the following effects of combining the drug and alcohol should the nurse include? Select all that apply.**

1. nausea and copious vomiting
2. severe flushing, headache, and vertigo
3. hypotension, chest pain, and syncope
4. somnolence progressing to coma

87. **When assessing the fetal heart rate with the nonstress test (NST) at 34 weeks, what type of accelerations should normally occur during a 20-minute period of observation?**

1. at least 2 accelerations of at least 20 bpm over 20 seconds
2. at least 2 accelerations of at least 15 bpm over 15 seconds
3. at least 1 acceleration of at least 10 bpm over 10 seconds
4. at least 1 acceleration of at least 5 bpm over 5 seconds

88. **Which metabolic effect is most common if a client is taking a loop diuretic?**

1. hypouricemia
2. hyperglycemia
3. hyperkalemia
4. hypokalemia

89. **An infant is to receive 65 milligrams of acetaminophen elixir every 4 to 6 hours as needed for fever. The elixir contains 80 milligrams per 5 milliliters. How many milliliters should be administered to equal 65 milligrams? Record your answer rounding to the nearest whole number.**

_____ milliliters.

90. **The nurse is caring for an elderly Hmong client who had a severe myocardial infarction and whose death appears imminent. Even though healthcare providers are still trying to save the client's life, family members are insisting that she be dressed in traditional clothing that they have brought from home. Which of the following is the most appropriate response?**

1. tell them that they cannot interrupt treatment
2. suggest they wait until efforts to save the client end
3. assist them to dress the client if possible
4. advise them that clothing is not important

91. A client receiving treatment for breast cancer feels severely anxious. Which of the following interventions are likely to be the most effective? Select all that apply.

1. instructing the client in relaxation exercises
2. encouraging the client to express concerns
3. advising the client that the anxiety will reduce in time
4. reminding the client that recovery rates are high
5. determining what relieves the client's anxiety

92. Which of the following are true regarding premature ventricular contractions? Select all that apply.

1. PVC's can be harmless abnormalities.
2. Frequent PVC's signify a myocardial infarction.
3. PVC's can occur in conjunction with underlying dysrhythmias.
4. PVC's can be caused by caffeine, nicotine or alcohol.

93. A client has terminal cancer. For months, the client's spouse has been teary and obviously grieving about the impending death, but now that death is imminent, the spouse seems detached and relatively unemotional. Which of the following is the most likely reason for the spouse's reaction?

1. lack of feelings for the spouse
2. state of emotional shock
3. dulling of responses because of substance abuse
4. premature completion of anticipatory grief

94. A client is receiving warfarin for venous thrombosis, and the client's INR is 4.0 with no evidence of bleeding. What action does the nurse anticipate?

1. administer warfarin as prescribed
2. administer increased dosage of warfarin until INR increases
3. hold or administer reduced dosage until INR decreases
4. hold warfarin and administer vitamin K orally

95. Which of the following is a common psychosocial response of a pregnant client to pregnancy during the first trimester?

1. increasing dependency
2. alteration in body image
3. ambivalence
4. changes in sexuality

96. A client with an inoperative brain tumor is expected to lapse into a coma. Place the usual stages in the continuum of states of consciousness (in Roman numerals) in descending order in the table below:

I. confusion
II. delirium
III. arousal
IV. vegetative state
V. stupor

Consciousness
Wakefulness
(1)
Drowsiness
(2)
Inattentiveness
(3)
(4)
(5)
Coma

97. Indicate the location of the right lumbar region (by letter) in the space below.

_____Right lumbar region

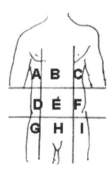

98. A patient with chronic glomerulonephritis has the following nursing diagnoses: activity intolerance, self-care deficit, excess fluid volume, ineffective self-health management, and anxiety. Considering Maslow's hierarchy of needs, which two of these needs should have priority?

1. excess fluid volume and anxiety
2. excess fluid volume and self-care deficit
3. excess fluid volume and activity intolerance
4. excess fluid volume and ineffective self-health management

99. A client in the psychiatric unit engages in yelling and name-calling with anger escalating, exhibiting the prodromal syndrome. The nurse is concerned that the client is at risk of self- or other-directed violence. Which of the following is the most appropriate initial intervention?

1. restrain the client
2. offer medication to relax client
3. attempt to talk the client down
4. call for additional help

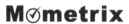

100. A client at a family planning clinic has received a prescription for oral contraceptives. When reviewing the client's medication list, the nurse notes that the client takes the following:

- St. John's wort 300 mg three times daily
- vitamin D3 500 mg daily
- calcium carbonate 1000 mg daily
- acetaminophen 650 mg every 6 hours as needed for headache
- multivitamin capsule daily

Which of the following information should the nurse include when educating the client about taking oral contraceptives?

1. these medications and supplements should not interfere with oral contraceptives
2. vitamin D3 and calcium carbonate should not be taken with oral contraceptives
3. St. John's wort may decrease the effectiveness of oral contraceptives
4. St. John's wort should not be taken with calcium carbonate or multivitamins

101. When assessing a neonate 's respiratory status, which of the following is an indication of respiratory distress. Select all that apply.

1. respiratory rate of 50 breaths per minute at rest
2. flaring nostrils
3. grunting expirations
4. sternal retraction
5. intercostal retractions

102. For which of the following reasons are benzodiazepines usually avoided in frail older adults?

1. may result in respiratory depression
2. may increase risk of falls
3. may increase risk of osteoporosis
4. may increase risk of hypertension

103. When reviewing dietary restrictions with an immunocompromised client following kidney transplantation, the client should be advised to avoid which of the following food products?

1. bean sprouts
2. strawberries
3. all citrus fruits
4. milk products

104. A client has been taking 112 micrograms of levothyroxine daily, but the physician has changed the dosage to 0.224 milligrams daily, and the patient wants to use up the tablets on hand. How many 112 microgram tablets equal 0.224 milligrams? Record your answer using a whole number.

_____ tablets

105. The first indication of amniotic fluid embolism (also called pregnancy-related anaphylactoid syndrome) is usually sudden onset of which of the following?

1. severe chest pain
2. acute dyspnea
3. hemorrhage
4. hypotension

106. A physician has prescribed nortriptyline hydrochloride, a tricyclic antidepressant, for a client with postherpetic syndrome who prefers not to take opioids because of a history of substance abuse. When discussing use of the drug with the client, which of the following information should the nurse include? Select all that apply.

1. the medication should be taken at bedtime
2. the medication must be taken with food
3. the client may need to take a stool softener
4. the client should report urinary dysfunction
5. the client may experience sexual dysfunction

107. Following an automobile accident that resulted in what appeared to be a mild head injury and fractured right clavicle, the client is being carefully monitored. The client's telemetry had shown a normal ECG complex with normal pulse rate until the following changes occurred:

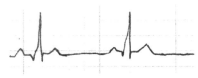

What does this tracing most likely represent?

1. sinus bradycardia resulting from increasing intracranial pressure
2. sinus bradycardia resulting from hypovolemia
3. premature ventricular contraction resulting from hypovolemia
4. premature ventricular contraction resulting from increasing intracranial pressure

108. A 2-year-old child is at the 25th percentile in height but the fourth percentile in weight. The child is slightly anemic, but other laboratory tests, including those for parasites and lead poisoning, are negative. Which of the following is the most likely next step?

1. identify food allergies/ restrictions
2. refer the child to Child Protective Services
3. observe the child's meal behaviors/practices
4. obtain a dietary intake history for the previous 24 hours and next 3 to 5 days

109. A client newly diagnosed with schizophrenia has been exhibiting both negative and positive symptoms. Which of the following symptoms would be categorized as negative?

1. inappropriate affect
2. visual hallucination
3. delusion of grandeur
4. disheveled appearance

110. A client has been diagnosed with end-stage kidney disease and is to begin hemodialysis at an outpatient dialysis center. Which of the following types of access is the best option for most clients?

1. venous catheter
2. AV graft
3. AV fistula
4. implanted port

111. A client has been diagnosed with amyotrophic lateral sclerosis (ALS) and uses a wheelchair, but still breathes independently. At what point may the client receive palliative care?

1. when the client becomes ventilator dependent or near death
2. when the client's life expectancy is 6 months or less
3. at any time since the client has a life-threatening disease
4. when the client is in need of pain control

112. Which of the following findings are consistent with early graft rejection in intestine recipients?

1. change in stool output
2. decreased hemoglobin and hematocrit
3. hypotension
4. decreased serum amylase

113. A client has had a long-leg plaster of Paris cast applied. What precautions should the nurse take to promote drying of the cast?

1. the cast should be covered with a blanket to increase heat
2. the cast should be left exposed and the client turned every 2 to 3 hours
3. the cast should be elevated on bolsters at the ankle to allow air to circulate
4. the cast should be dried manually with a hair dryer set on high heat

114. A patient presents in a deep coma with decorticate posturing, which suggests damage to which part of the brain?

1. midbrain
2. right and left hemispheres
3. medulla
4. diencephalon

115. A client who has been taking digoxin presents in the emergency department with an irregular pulse and bradycardia of 22 to 28 bpm as well as nausea, vomiting, diarrhea, headache, and halo vision. Which of the following interventions does the nurse anticipate? Select all that apply.

1. administer an increased dose of digoxin
2. administer digoxin immune Fab
3. administer atropine
4. provide supportive treatment
5. conduct laboratory tests for digoxin and electrolyte levels
6. carry out continuous cardiac monitoring

116. Two months following allogenic hematopoietic cell transplantation, a client has increasing diarrhea, a red rash over parts of the body, and severe generalized itching; the client's sclerae appear slightly yellow tinged. Which of the following disorders does the nurse suspect?

1. allergic response to anti-rejection drugs
2. acute graft vs host disease
3. liver failure
4. chronic graft vs host disease

117. When a client is terminally ill and in the end stages of life, decisions about treatment options, such as whether to provide rehydration, should be based on which of the following considerations?

1. alleviating symptoms that may cause family distress
2. prolonging the client's life as long as possible
3. following standard protocols for end-of-life care
4. providing comfort and honoring client's wishes

118. A patient with interstitial cystitis has been prescribed home bladder instillations with an anesthetic (lidocaine) mixture but has not been doing the instillations consistently because the instillation causes severe burning when she urinates to empty the instillation from the bladder after the prescribed period. Which of the following is likely the best solution?

1. discontinue instillations
2. clamp the catheter for the prescribed period and then open to drain fluid before removal
3. remove the catheter after instillation and then insert a second catheter to drain the bladder
4. take an analgesic prior to the instillation

119. A client with Hodgkin's disease has severe pruritus that prevents him from sleeping and causes him considerable discomfort. Which of the following measures may be most effective in relieving itching? Select all that apply.

1. maintaining room humidity at 50% to 60% and temperature at 70°F to 72°F
2. taking diphenhydramine as needed
3. taking opioid medications
4. taking oatmeal baths
5. taking barbiturates

120. The nurse has obtained a unit of packed red blood cells that is to be administered to a client with leukemia. Within how many minutes must the transfusion be initiated after removal from the blood bank refrigerator?

1. 15 minutes
2. 30 minutes
3. 45 minutes
4. 60 minutes

Answer Key and Explanations for Test #3

1. 3: Both foam overlays and sheepskin are inappropriate for incontinent clients. The alternating pressure overlay is the best choice because it is liquid-resistant and has cells or cylinders that alternately inflate and deflate at intervals, controlled by a pump. They should only be used with clients <250 pounds, so the client fits this criterion. While the low air loss bed provides a superior support surface, it is much more expensive and must be monitored carefully and maintained properly, and it can result in hypothermia because of the constant flow of air.

2. 30: The problem can be calculated using dimensional analysis:

$$\frac{120 \; mL}{1 \; hour} \times \frac{15 \; drops}{1 \; mL} \times \frac{1 \; hour}{60 \; min}$$

Eliminate like terms (mL and hour) and reduce 120/60:

$$\frac{2}{1} \times \frac{15 \; drops}{1} \times \frac{1}{1 \; min} = 30 \; \frac{drops}{min}$$

3. 2: The 3-point gait requires the client to have the most upper body strength and balance because the client must support the entire weight of the body with the arms. The sequence for ambulation is to start with both feet together and the crutch tips slightly to the front and side of the feet. Then, the client advances the weaker leg and both crutches at the same time with the toe even with the crutches, followed by the stronger leg with the toe advancing slightly past the crutches. Note: the crutches are advanced only with the weaker leg.

4. 2, 4, and 5: The nurse should cover the client with a warm blanket, leaving the cast exposed to the air so that it can dry properly. The client should be turned and repositioned every 2 to 3 hours so that all sides of the cast can dry evenly. While some facilities use heat cradles or commercial cast dryers at low temperatures, high-powered electric fans should not blow directly on the cast as this may result in the outside drying and the inside remaining damp. Fans may be used away from the cast to increase air circulation in the room.

5. 1: While protocols regarding tube feedings may vary somewhat, generally if gastric residual is less than 100 mL, it is returned to the stomach and the tubing flushed with 30 mL of water, but if it is more than 100mL (in this case 150 mL) it may indicate that an obstruction has occurred, and the nurse should hold the feeding and notify the MD before proceeding. The amount of residual gastric contents should be aspirated and measured at least every 8 hours.

6. 0.25: To complete the calculation, first convert micrograms to milligrams: 50 mcg = 0.05 mg.

$$\text{Tablets needed} = \frac{\text{desired dose}}{\text{available dose}}$$

$$\frac{0.05}{0.2} = 0.25 \; tablets$$

7. 1, 2, and 3: Difficulty urinating is a common problem after surgery, and conservative methods should be tried before catheterization. Methods to promote urination include pouring warm water over the client's perineum, asking the client to blow bubbles through a straw into a glass of water, and turning on running water while the client attempts to urinate. Telling a client to "just relax" may increase stress. It's more helpful to lead the client through relaxation exercises.

8. 3, 4, and 5: The irrigating syringe should be filled with about 50 mL of irrigant but it should be instilled slowly, using care not to occlude the ear canal with the syringe tip as this may result in increased pressure and rupture of the eardrum. The client should be positioned lying flat or sitting with the head turned toward the affected ear to facilitate drainage and help secure the drainage basin. On those over 3 years old, the pinna is pulled up and back. The solution should drain out freely during the irrigation.

9. 1: Acupuncture has been demonstrated to relieve chemotherapy-induced nausea and vomiting in a number of studies. Some studies also seem to indicate that ginger (usually in tea form) can reduce the intensity of nausea but not vomiting. The nurse may recommend both of these therapies. However, there is no evidence to suggest that therapeutic touch or magnetic therapy are effective in relieving nausea, and herbal therapies must be evaluated individually as some may interact negatively with the client's medications.

10. 1: While pain is usually considered to be that which the client states it is, the one-to-ten scale that is commonly used in the United States is not always used in other countries. People from Hispanic countries often describe pain in terms of small amount, normal, or strong. The nurse should use a different type of questioning to ascertain pain and might state, "I see that you are rubbing your stomach and seem to be in pain" to encourage dialogue.

11. 3: If a client in cervical traction complains of increasing pain in the jaw and ears, the chinstrap may be exerting excess pull on the chin, resulting in increased pressure on the temporomandibular joint. The nurse should gently correct the client's head position by tilting the head slightly forward to relieve the pull on the chin. If the pain occurs on only one side, then the traction may be uneven, and the client's body may need to be positioned correctly.

12. 2: When taking a verbal order of any kind, including a telephone order, the nurse should write the order and then read it back, asking for verbal verification that the order is correct, before notifying the pharmacy of the order or administering the medication. In an emergency situation only, such as may occur with a cardiac arrest, the nurse may repeat back an order for verification. Verbal orders should not be accepted if the physician is present on the unit.

13. 2: Unless the client is in danger, the nurse should not confront the nurse he suspects of taking an opioid medication intended for a client, because a confrontation may end badly. The other nurse may deny the accusation and place blame on the first nurse or may even react violently. Instead, the observing nurse should immediately notify a supervisor of his concerns so that the administration can carry out an investigation according to facility protocol, which also determines whether an incident report needs to be completed.

14. 2: While state laws vary regarding how to report and what to report, all states require mandatory reporting of suspected child abuse. Because the type and extent of injuries to the child are not consistent with a fall off of a swing and the child has evidence of multiple previous injuries, the incident must be reported to the proper authorities. In most states, the report is made to Child Protective Services, who in turn may notify the police.

15. 4: The most appropriate response to a client's complaint is to express empathy and gather information without placing blame or making excuses: "I'm so sorry you felt that way. Can you tell me what happened?" Allowing a client to ventilate feelings is often sufficient, but if the issue is serious, the nurse should describe the client's response to the nurse involved and then follow the same procedures in listening to the nurse in order to try to reach a resolution.

16. 3 and 5: Decimal numbers should contain a leading zero, such as with "0.5% albuterol inhalation solution." If the zero is missing, such as with ".25 mg budesonide inhalation solution," the initial period may be overlooked or read as a number one and the statement misread as "25 mg" or "125 mg." Similarly, trailing zeroes should be avoided after whole numbers, "10 mg" instead of "10.0 mg." Abbreviations such as "SOB," which may be misinterpreted as a pejorative or as "short of breath" or "side of bed" should also be avoided and the words written out.

17. 2: If the neonate swallowed amniotic fluid, the child may be born in acute respiratory distress, but symptoms may be delayed for a few hours, so the child must be monitored carefully. If the neonate cries at delivery and shows no signs of distress, then the mouth and throat are suctioned, but if respiratory distress is evident, the child should be intubated and tracheobronchial suctioning done to remove meconium plugs. The gastric contents may be suctioned as well to prevent the infant from regurgitating and aspirating meconium.

18. 2: Two forms of identifiers should always be used prior to administering medication to any client, even if the nurse recognizes the client and is relatively sure of the client's identity. Asking the client's name and checking the hospital ID bracelet meet minimal requirements. In some cases, clients may be identified by asking their names and birthdates. The nurse should always double check the name on the medication as well. An ID bracelet that is not on the client but elsewhere, such as on a bedside stand, should not be used for identification.

19. 4: While a gait/transfer belt may be used by a caregiver until the client is independent, a sliding board is most indicated because the client cannot stand and requires sitting transfer. Use is quite simple and sliding boards are relatively inexpensive. They are usually made of rigid plastic material with low friction so that the client can easily slide from the chair onto the toilet or another surface. Any caregiver who will be assisting should be instructed in methods to use to assist the client without causing injury to the caregiver or the client.

20. 2: According to OSHA guidelines, if items are out of reach, the acceptable work practice is to get a properly maintained ladder and use that to climb up to reach the objects. The nurse should never use stools, chairs, or boxes in place of a ladder or try to "climb" up a cabinet by standing on a lower shelf. It's important to climb high enough on the ladder that the nurse is not lifting items over the head because this can result in injuries and falls.

21. 3:

This is the international symbol for biohazards. Biohazards are biological materials (plants, animals, organisms), such as bacteria, viruses, and parasites, which are dangerous to people's health or pose the risk of infection. In medical facilities, items that must be labeled as biohazards include used hypodermic needles and contaminated dressings because they may contain infectious biological material. Each facility should establish protocols for handling and disposing of biohazardous materials. Biohazardous waste products are generally disposed of in red plastic bags with the biohazard symbol on the bag.

22. 1, 2, 4, and 5: The client should dispose of syringes and needles in a sharps disposal container (or glass jar) immediately after use, being sure to maintain the container out of reach of children and pets. The container should be disposed of when it is about three-quarters full because if the container is too full, the risk of accidental puncture increases. While the container may be disposed of in the regular trash in some areas, other areas are more restrictive, so the client must check with the local community garbage disposal company for guidelines. Needles should never be flushed down the toilet.

23. 2: Because attempting to evacuate clients from the facility is likely to increase exposure to the hazardous material, the most likely emergency response is to shelter in place. This applies to both staff and clients. Guidelines may vary according to the type of waste but can include locking doors, sealing doors and windows, and shutting off air-conditioning and forced-air systems. Many facilities have windows that do not open, but if not, windows should be closed immediately. Staff should monitor news reports because emergency personnel may not be readily available to provide information.

24. 2, 3, 4, and 6: Clients with gastrointestinal disorders and diarrhea should be maintained on both standard precautions and contact precautions. The nurse should use personal protective equipment (gown and gloves) for all contact with the client but does not need to wear a mask or N95 respirator. The client should be in a private room or ≥3 feet away from other clients. Because *C. difficile* spreads readily, special care must be taken with environmental cleaning. Nurses should wash hands with soap and water rather than alcohol antiseptic and should avoid sharing electronic thermometers used by the client with others.

25. 125 mg: Because the child is to receive 25 mg for each kilogram of weight, the calculation is to simply multiply 25 X 10 = 250 mg. Since the total dosage is to be given in two divided doses, the nurse will administer 125 mg (250/2) at each dose.

26. 2: The Safe Babies® apron is a one-piece apron that fits over the head and attaches on the side with Velcro closures. The apron contains two large pockets in the front and two in the back, so the nurse can carry 4 infants at one time. Infants should be wrapped in blankets for warmth prior to being placed in the pockets. The apron is designed so the person's arms are free. This allows the nurse to carry supplies or even additional infants if necessary.

27. 4: Because this is an emergency situation, the nurse should immediately obtain a second ECG machine and conduct the ECG. This may involve sending another staff member to a different unit, but the nurse should remain with the client. Once finished, the nurse should label the first machine as "Out of Order" and follow facility procedures for initiating repairs. Under no circumstances should the nurse use equipment that is damaged and may cause a spark because of the danger this poses to the clients and staff.

28. 2: Because nurses work closely with clients, a client often divulges confidential information, such as the fact that she has been having an affair with her husband's brother. However, the nurse must evaluate communications to determine if they are health related and can and should be reported or if they are private communications. In this case, no purpose is served by reporting the client's statement except to spread gossip, so this is a HIPAA violation of privacy.

29. 2: If at all possible, each treatment should be documented immediately after completion. Treatments should never be documented in advance, even if they are routine and the nurse is relatively sure they will be completed. The longer the period of time following completion of a treatment, the greater the chance that an error in documenting (such as forgetting to chart) will occur. If the nurse cannot document immediately, then the nurse should make a note of the time and essential information. Documenting should not be left until the end of shift.

30. 3: The most helpful information for the homeless client is probably a list of shelters and community agencies, especially those with programs to assist the homeless. Adult Protective Services investigates abuse, but cuts resulting from a fight are not usually considered abusive situations. Many homeless people are very reluctant to deal with the police in any way. Providing a list of 12-step organizations is not indicated unless the client is inebriated or there is other evidence of a drinking problem.

31. 1: If a nurse believes that current procedures should be changed, then the best place to begin is with a survey of the literature regarding wound care to determine what best practices are recommended. Armed with this information, the nurse can approach the director of nursing or other appropriate person and discuss other methods, such as interviews and questionnaires, which might help to determine the need for change, those interested in assisting, and the best way to proceed.

32. 4: The best approach is "What do you understand about your options for care?" The nurse should never suggest that treatment won't help because even those in hospice and palliative care receive treatment. However, the focus of treatment is different, so the nurse should stress that the goal of hospice and palliative care is to keep the client as comfortable as possible. Clients may feel they are being abandoned if the nurse suggests stopping all treatments.

33. 1, 2, 3, and 5: Clients who have undergone gastric bypass surgery should avoid concentrated sugars as they accelerate emptying of the stomach. Clients should drink liquids at least 30 minutes before meals rather than with foods and should eat 5 or 6 small meals a day rather than 3 large meals. Dairy products should be restricted to low-fat products, but many people find dairy products cause diarrhea, so they should be introduced cautiously. Those with dumping syndrome may find that reclining after eating slows emptying of the stomach and reduces symptoms.

34. 4: A Durable Power of Attorney for Healthcare remains in effect (durable) if the client is unable to make decisions, so this is the best option. While state laws vary somewhat, a Durable Power of Attorney for Healthcare is generally limited to healthcare decisions only. In some states, a healthcare proxy can be established as part of an Advance Directive, but in other states two different documents are required, so the nurse should always be familiar with state regulations.

35. 1, 3, and 4: Rear-facing car seats are safest, and neonates should always be placed in rear-facing seats. Car seats should be secured in the middle of the back seat, away from airbags, or airbags should be disconnected. Neonates are at risk for hypoxia in car seats, so the parents should ensure the child's neck is straight, avoiding the chin-to-chest position, and should limit time in the car seat to short trips of ≤60 minutes. Harnesses should be secure so that only one finger can easily slide underneath. No car seat involved in an accident should be used again even if no damage is evident.

36. 2: While some children with pinworms (*Enterobius vermicularis*) may be essentially asymptomatic, common findings include intense anal itching and vulvovaginitis in girls. Those infected often are restless at night and sleep poorly and may complain of intermittent abdominal pain and nausea. The tape test (tape across the anus at bedtime) is the most common diagnostic procedure because the mature worms crawl through the anus to lay eggs in the perineal folds and become attached to the tape.

37. 1: Providing basic care but refusing to talk to the client is a violation of provision 1 of the ANA Code of Ethics for Nurses. This provision requires that the nurse practice with compassion and show respect for each individual, regardless of social/economic status, personal attributes, or type of health problems. It's the nurse's responsibility to provide care to the highest standard to all patients. Attempting to avoid caring for a particular client does not violate the Code of Ethics but it may be construed as unprofessional.

38. 3: Even if hospital policy allows nurses to avoid caring for clients undergoing abortions, this does not excuse the nurse from the ethical responsibility of attending to emergency situations, such as the possibility that the client is hemorrhaging. The nurse should immediately evaluate the client to determine whether emergency intervention is needed. If so, the nurse should follow protocol; if not, the nurse should reassure the client and notify the client's nurse when he or she returns.

39. 3: While most immunizations of infants begin at 6 to 8 weeks, the hepatitis B vaccine should be administered within 12 hours of birth to all infants because hepatitis B is transmitted through body fluids and can be contracted during birth. A series of three injections of monovalent HepB are required, with the second injection between one and two months and the third at or after 24 weeks. If the mother tests positive for hepatitis B, then the infant should be given both the monovalent HepB vaccination as well as HepB immune globulin within 12 hours of birth.

40. 2, 3, and 4: Positive reinforcement provides something in return for a change in behavior. This can include tangible rewards, such as an additional hour of Internet use or some type of privilege, or supportive statements, such as "You are making good progress." Sometimes positive reinforcement occurs naturally as a result of behavioral change, such as when the client gains one-half pound. When possible, positive reinforcement should occur immediately after a behavioral change so that the client makes a positive association with the behavior.

41. 4: Intramuscular (IM) injections are almost always given to adults with a needle that is 1.5 inches in length. A shorter length (1 inch) should be reserved for children or for very thin adults. The needle gauge usually varies from 21 to 25, although very thick preparations may require a gauge of 18 or 19. IM injections are usually given with a 3-mL syringe, although the maximum amount of medication in each injection should not exceed 2 mL. If larger volumes are ordered, then the dose should be divided and administered in two injections.

42. 1, 3, and 5: As clients age, their pulmonary elasticity tends to decrease while their chest-wall rigidity increases, making it more difficult to adequately ventilate. Pharyngeal reflexes, which serve a protective role in preventing choking and aspiration, also decrease. Alveoli become distended, decreasing alveolar surface area, and there is ventilation/perfusion mismatching, impairing the exchange of oxygen. Older adults undergoing surgery may need extended preoxygenation prior to surgery and higher concentrations of oxygen during the procedure to avoid hypoxia.

43. 2: Current guidelines advise women ages 40 to 64 to have Pap smears every two to three years. If Pap smears have been negative for three consecutive years, then many physicians recommend three-year intervals; however, pelvic exams may be done more frequently to assess for other abnormalities or disorders, such as chlamydia or other sexually transmitted diseases. Women who have undergone a total hysterectomy may be advised that they no longer need Pap smears because of removal of the cervix.

44. 1, 2, 3, and 4: The Centers for Disease Control (CDC) recommendations for immunizations for adults older than age 65 include annual influenza vaccinations. The client should receive a pneumococcal vaccination if he has not been previously vaccinated. There are two different types of pneumococcal vaccination: PPSV23 is recommended for those 65 and older, but PCV13 may be recommended according to risk factors as well. Clients should receive a tetanus-diphtheria booster every 10 years. The herpes zoster vaccination is recommended one time for those 60 and older. High-risk clients may be advised to have additional vaccinations.

45. 1: Breast cancer results in more deaths in women ages 15 to 34 and 35 to 54 than any other type of cancer. However, younger women have lower rates of breast cancer. Survival rates are lower for women with an onset of breast cancer prior to age 40 because the cancers tend to be more aggressive and screening tools are less effective for younger women because of the density of the breast tissue, making early diagnosis more difficult.

46. 1: The ethical principle of autonomy recognizes that clients have the right to make their own informed decisions about their care. The most important assessment is of the client's cognitive ability because the client needs to be able to understand and consider information that is given by healthcare providers. Children may be able to make informed decisions, but the law does not allow them to do so unless they are emancipated, so the right of autonomy passes to the parents or guardians. Likewise, clients who have cognitive impairment may not be able to make informed decisions.

47. 2: Vitamin B$_9$ (folic acid/folate) is necessary to prevent neural tube defects. These defects of the brain, spinal cord, and/or spine occur within the first month of pregnancy, so women who are planning a pregnancy should begin taking the vitamin prior to becoming pregnant and then continue taking the vitamin throughout pregnancy. Most multivitamins contain folic acid, and it may also be included in enriched cereals. Dietary sources of folate (the naturally occurring form) include dark-green leafy vegetables such as spinach, mustard greens, and collard greens as well as beets, broccoli, lentils, and other beans.

48. 3: The normal fetal heart rate (FHR) at term is 120 to 160, with rates lower than 120 being considered bradycardia and greater than 160 being considered tachycardia. The FHR at 5 weeks is usually in the 80s, increasing each day by about 3 beats over the next month. By week 9 of gestation, the FHR has increased to about 175 and ranges from 120 to 180 by midpregnancy. However, the FHR tends to slow somewhat during the last 10 weeks.

49. 2, 4, and 6: Braxton Hicks contractions (false labor) begin at about six weeks of gestation and continue sporadically throughout pregnancy. Braxton Hicks contractions may be difficult to differentiate from true labor as the mother nears term, but they are characterized by contractions with no associated dilation of the cervix. Discomfort is usually felt in the lower abdomen rather than over the uterine fundus, and it does not radiate. Contractions may become rhythmic but do not become longer in duration or at closer intervals, and they may resolve with ambulation or pain medication.

50. 2: The Apgar test is given at one minute and five minutes after birth to determine if emergency care is needed. A total score of ≥7 is a sign of good health.

Sign	0	1	2
Appearance (skin color)	Cyanosis or pallor over entire body	Normal, except for extremities	Entire body is normal
Pulse (heart rate)	Absent	<100 bpm	>100 bpm
Grimace (reflex irritability)	Unresponsive	Grimace	Infant sneezes, coughs, and recoils
Activity (muscle tone)	Absent	Flexed extremities	Infant moves freely
Respiration (breathing rate and effort)	Absent	Bradypnea, dyspnea	Good breathing and crying

51. 2: The best response to the client who believes she does not need RhoGAM with a first pregnancy is the one that provides a reason why the treatment is needed: "You need treatment during your first pregnancy to prevent Rh incompatibility reactions during a second pregnancy." The serum RhoGAM contains Rh+ antibodies that agglutinate any stray fetal red blood cells that enter the mother's bloodstream to prevent antibodies forming against them because these antibodies can attack a future fetus. The mother receives RhoGAM at 26 to 28 weeks and again within 72 hours of delivery.

52. 2, 4, and 5: Latex condoms should be used one time only for each act of oral, vaginal, or anal sex and should be used only with water-based lubricants because oil-based lubricants may cause deterioration of the latex. Room should be left at the tip of the condom for sperm to collect. Latex condoms should not be used with nonoxynol-9 because this increases the risk of transmission of HIV and STDs. Condoms should be removed immediately after ejaculation before the penis becomes flaccid. No contraceptive device provides 100% protection against pregnancy, HIV, and STDs.

53. 2, 3, 4, and 5: The purpose of personal protective equipment (PPE) is to protect the wearer against hazards in the workplace, so the equipment may vary from one workplace to another. Goggles, respirators, masks, gloves, and gowns are commonly used PPE in nursing, but personal radiation dosimeters may also be considered as PPE if the nurse is exposed to radiation in the workplace and needs to monitor the exposure. Back belts have not been shown in studies to reduce the risk of back injuries, are not considered PPE, and are not recommended for use.

54. 2: The client must see a physician immediately because she is at risk for rabies; most cases of rabies in the United States are traced to infections from bats. Most bats that humans are able to approach are ill, increasing the danger. Rabies prophylaxis must be given before the onset of neurological symptoms, so the nurse should stress that the client should not wait to see if symptoms occur because, once she develops rabies, death is almost certain.

55. 4: The best response is "Would you like information about community programs available to help you be safer?" because it is neither judgmental nor pitying and doesn't try to impose a course of action that the client may be unwilling to accept, but it does allow the client to have a choice. Nurses often hear information from clients that is surprising or even shocking, and it's important to deal with this information in a very professional, matter-of-fact manner.

56. 3: The nurse should avoid using the dorsogluteal site in obese adults because adipose tissue may make it difficult to inject into the muscle. Generally, this site should be avoided if at all possible in all clients because of the danger of hitting the sciatic nerve. The deltoid muscle should be used only for small volumes of medication. The preferred site for intramuscular (IM) injections is the

111

ventrogluteal site. When giving an IM injection in the vastus lateralis site, the tissue must be pinched and the muscle should be pulled away rather than the skin being held taut. This site is preferred for children younger than 18 months of age.

57: The first action when any type of adverse reaction occurs with a transfusion is to immediately stop the transfusion.

Order of actions:

1: (First) II. Stop the transfusion.
2: (Second) I. Notify the physician.
3: (Third) III. Notify the blood bank.
4: (Fourth) IV. Administer medications (usually antihistamine) as ordered.

This type of reaction is classified as a mild to moderate allergic response and may occur during the transfusion and up to an hour after completion of the transfusion and is generally caused by an allergy to a residual plasma protein in the donor's blood.

58. 2.5 mL. Calculation:

50 (mg)/1 (mL) = 125 (mg)/x (mL).
50 × x = 50x.
1 × 125 = 125.
50x = 125.
125/50 = 2.5 mL.

59. 2: After insertion of a Foley catheter into a male client, his penis should be positioned upward so that the catheter doesn't catch on his legs, and it should be secured by tape to the right or left lower abdomen, with the tubing looped so the client has slack to turn from side to side, and then the tube is taped to the edge of the bed. The tubing should hang vertically down from the mattress to the collection bag so the urine drains properly.

60. 2: Clients taking oral contraceptives should be advised to avoid smoking because smoking increases the risk of clot formation, which can result in heart attacks or strokes. The risk is especially high after age 35, but all women who smoke should consider an alternate method of birth control. Alcohol and diet do not increase health risks with contraceptives, although alcohol may have other negative effects. There is some evidence that women taking oral contraceptives have more muscle tenderness after exercise, but there is no increased health risk.

61. Correct order:

1. V. Raise the head of the bed to 30° with the client in the supine position.
2. III. Place the client's upper arm across her chest and roll her to a side-lying position toward the nurse by pulling and supporting her shoulders and hips.
3. IV. Place one arm under the client's shoulders, supporting her head and neck, and place the other arm over her thighs.
4. II. Pivot the client by moving her legs over the side of the bed and elevating her trunk.
5. I. Support the client until she is stable.

62. 3: Knots should always be free of the pulleys with any type of traction because if the knot lodges in the pulley, it may interfere with the line of pull, which should be along the bone axis, with the weights hanging freely. The tension rope should be in the groove of the pulley and should slide easily. The nurse should ensure that the client is lying centered on the bed because if the client's body is not aligned properly with the traction, then the line of pull may be altered.

63. Correct order:

1. V. Wash hands and apply gloves.
2. I. Open the plug on the port.
3. II. Open the Hemovac over the container, and tilt the port toward the container so the fluid drains into the container.
4. IV. Cleanse the plug and the port with an alcohol wipe in the dominant hand while compressing and holding the top and bottom of the Hemovac together with the other hand.
5. III. Place the plug into the port.

64. 30 minutes: Administration of medications through an NG tube under suction should be avoided if possible because some of the medication may be suctioned out; however, if medication is ordered, the nurse must disconnect the suction prior to administration, ensure the NG tube is properly placed (injecting air and listening for gurgling, aspirating, and checking the pH), flush the NG tube with 30 mL water, administer the medication, flush the tubing with another 30 mL water, and leave it disconnected from the suction for 30 minutes to allow time for the medication to be absorbed.

65. 2: Temperatures for hot and cold applications:

- Hot: 37 to 41° C/98 to 106° F.
- Warm: 34 to 37° C/93 to 98° F.
- Lukewarm: 26 to 34° C/80 to 93° F.
- Cool: 18 to 26° C/65 to 80° F.
- Cold: 10 to 18° C/50 to 65° F.

Hot and cold applications should be limited to durations of 10 to 20 minutes because longer periods may result in tissue damage. Because moisture conducts heat, hot compresses increase the risk of burns.

66. 1, 3, and 6: Cold applications block peripheral nerve conduction and provide local anesthesia, so cold may be used to reduce pain. Cold increases the viscosity of the blood, promoting coagulation at a site of injury. Cold also results in vasoconstriction, which reduces edema and inflammation; decreased muscle tension, which helps to prevent muscle spasms; and reduced cell metabolism. Heat applications tend to have the opposite effect, resulting in vasodilation, decreased viscosity of the blood, increased permeability of capillaries, and increased tissue metabolism.

67. 2: The integrity of the closed system of drainage should be maintained. The correct procedure for collecting a urine specimen from a self-sealing rubber catheter is to withdraw urine directly from the catheter by using a 20-mL (for urinalysis) or 3-mL (for culture) syringe with a 1-inch, 21-gauge needle. After cleansing the catheter with a disinfectant, the nurse inserts the needle at a 45-degree angle into the catheter near where it attaches to the drainage tube. After the urine is collected, it is injected into a sterile specimen container.

68. 1, 2, 5, and 6: To control exposure to dust mites, the nurse should advise the parents to keep the house clean and free of obvious dust and clutter, vacuuming frequently. They should encase the child's mattress and box spring in allergen-proof covers and wash the bed linens, pillows, clothing, and stuffed toys in hot water (>130°F) weekly. Humidity should be maintained below 50% with a dehumidifier. It is not essential that all carpets and upholstered furniture in the home be removed, but removing these from the child's bedroom will help to decrease exposure.

69. 3: The "spooning" position, in which the female and her partner are lying on their sides with the male behind the female, allows penetration without undue strain on either the male or the female. The nurse should also encourage them to engage in sexual activities during the times of day when they have less pain. Taking a warm bath prior to sexual activity may also help to reduce muscle stiffness and discomfort. Intimacy is important at all ages, and the nurse should discuss the matter openly with older clients.

70. 4: As Alzheimer's disease progresses, hallucinations, delusions, and "living in the past" are very common, and trying to convince clients that what they believe is not true can often result in frustration and aggressive behavior. If the hallucinations and delusions are benign and happy memories, the nurse should allow clients to believe them and not interfere. However, if they are frightening or upsetting to the clients, then the nurse should attempt to distract the clients and refocus their attention.

71. 1: Hypotension with narrowing pulse pressure, pulsus paradoxus, distant heart sounds, restlessness, bulging neck veins, and increasing cyanosis are indications of cardiac tamponade resulting from perforation of the ventricle and bleeding into the pericardial sac. This is a medical emergency, and the nurse must immediately notify the physician and prepare the client for surgery. Although nonhemorrhagic tamponade will usually respond well to pericardiocentesis, hemorrhagic tamponade requires thoracotomy because the bleeding will continue until its cause is corrected.

72. Order:

Enzyme/Protein	Rise	Peak	Return to normal
(1) IV. Myoglobin	2 hours	4 hours	24 hours
(2) II. CK-MB	4–8 hours	20 hours	≤72 hours
(3) III. Troponin I	3–6 hours	14–20 hours	5 to 7 days
(4) I. Troponin T	3–6 hours	12–24 hours	10 to 15 days

73. 1, 2, and 6: Raynaud's disease, intermittent digital arteriolar vasoconstriction, affects the hands and feet and may, with severe vasoconstriction, result in ulceration or gangrene. Vasoconstriction occurs with exposure to cold or stress and is exacerbated by smoking and some medications, so clients should be advised to quit smoking and avoid beta blockers and birth control pills. Clients should avoid the cold and wear gloves or mittens whenever exposed to cold temperatures or when handling cold or frozen foods. Treatment may include vasodilators and calcium channel blockers (nifedipine) and sympathectomy.

74. 4:

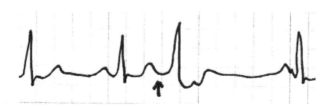

This ECG recording represents premature ventricular contraction (PVC). PVCs are ectopic beats that can occur early in otherwise healthy individuals, although they are of concern in those with preexisting heart disease because they may indicate a risk for more severe ventricular arrhythmias, such as ventricular tachycardia. The impulse for the ectopic beat originates within the ventricles prior to the sinus impulse. PVCs may occur singly or in pairs or in a recurring pattern and are often followed by a compensatory pause.

75. 64 mm Hg: The pulse pressure is the difference between the systolic blood pressure and the diastolic blood pressure:

156 – 92 = 64.

The normal range for the pulse pressure is 30 to 40. A narrow pulse pressure (<25% of systolic reading) indicates decreased left ventricular stroke volume and can also indicate decreased cardiac output, heart failure, or shock. A widened pulse pressure may indicate a number of different conditions, including atherosclerosis, arteriovenous fistula, thyrotoxicosis, heart block, endocarditis, and pregnancy.

76. 2: Brain tumors or traumatic brain injuries to different parts of the brain can result in specific types of symptoms:

- Frontal lobe: Changes in mood and personality as well as hemiparesis.
- Occipital lobe: Visual disturbances and visual hallucinations.
- Temporal lobe: Loss of memory, speech abnormalities, and lack of coordination.
- Parietal lobe: Loss of sensation; difficulty with fine motor skills, such as writing; and loss of half-body awareness.
- Cerebellum: Lack of balance and coordination.
- Brain stem: Dysphagia, facial pain, weakness, and cranial nerve dysfunction.

77. 3: Coma. The Glasgow Coma Scale (GCS) is based on scores assigned for three parameters: eye-opening response, verbal response, and muscle response. Scores range from 3 (worst possible) to 15 (best possible). Head injuries are classified according to the following scores:

- Coma—GCS score of 3 to 8.
- Severe head injury—GCS score of 8 or less.
- Moderate head injury—GCS score of 9 to 12.
- Mild head injury—GCS score of 13 to 15.

78. Correct order:

1. I. Six-hour postoperative client is asking for pain medication for pain of 8 on a scale of 1 to 10.
2. IV. Three-day postoperative client needs assessment for sudden elevated temperature.
3. III. Five-day postoperative client needs intermittent tube feeding.
4. II. Two-day postoperative client needs routine dressing change.

Acute needs are handled first (pain medication and evaluation). Because a routine dressing change is not time sensitive and tube feedings are given on a regular schedule (usually every four to six hours), the tube feeding should be done before the dressing change.

79. 2: An impaired nurse should not under any circumstances be allowed to care for clients. Nor should nurse A attempt to cover for the impaired nurse by observing her or assisting her with client care. Nurse A should immediately notify a supervisor of the concerns about nurse B. Confronting another nurse about substance abuse could result in denials or even a violent confrontation, so nurse A should not attempt to handle the situation independently.

80. 4: Tardive dyskinesia (TD) is a chronic adverse effect associated with haloperidol and other neuroleptic drugs as well as anticholinergics and substances of abuse. Elderly clients and those with schizophrenia and other neuropsychiatric diseases have an increased risk of developing TD, so these drugs should be used with care or avoided. Once symptoms develop, up to 50% of clients remain afflicted, even if the medication is discontinued. No established treatment is available, although different approaches can be tried, including herbal medicines.

81. 4: The glucose is high normal, but both kidney function tests, the BUN and serum creatinine, are markedly elevated, indicating probable kidney failure, so further testing for kidney disease is indicated.

Test	Result	Normal value
BUN	172 mg/dL	7-17 mg/dL
Serum creatinine	16.4 mg/dL	8.4-10.2 mg/dL
Glucose	98 mg/dL	70-99 mg/dL

82. 3: If a client is to receive two oral medications (capsules) per the enteral feeding tube, the nurse should open the capsules separately and dilute each with water. They should be drawn up in separate syringes for instilling. If the client has continuous feeding, the feeding should be stopped and the tube flushed with about 15 mL of water before instilling the first drug and then flushed again with the same volume after instillation to empty the tube of the medication before the second drug instillation. Then, the tube is flushed again before restarting the feeding.

83. 1, 2, 3, and 6: Age changes that typically occur in the respiratory system include blunting of the cough and laryngeal reflexes, making it harder to clear the lung to expel debris. Alveoli decrease in number but increase in size, making them less efficient at oxygen exchange. Ciliary action decreases, increasing the risk of pneumonia. The lungs lose elasticity and the thoracic muscles have increased rigidity. Overall, the lungs become smaller in size and have less ability to expand or expel debris. Residual volume tends to increase, so vital capacity decreases.

84. 1: When assessing a client's health history regarding intake of alcohol, the male client who goes out with friends 1 or 2 times a week and has 4 to 6 drinks each time would qualify as a person who is an "at-risk" drinker because he routinely drinks 4 or more drinks per occasion even though he is within the acceptable drinking range of up to 14 drinks (2 daily) per week. Females, because of differences in size and metabolism, should restrict drinking to no more than 1 drink per day.

85. 3: If 2 years after the death of her spouse, a client remains preoccupied with memories of her deceased husband, neglecting family and friends, the type of grief response the client is experiencing is prolonged. Prolonged grief may persist for many years after a death and may seriously impact a person's ability to function. Some who experience prolonged grief become suicidal. Exposure therapy, reliving and talking about the death, can help to relieve prolonged grief.

86. 1, 2, and 3: Disulfiram is a drug that alters the metabolism of alcohol, causing the level of acetaldehyde to increase markedly. This causes flushing, headache, and vertigo within minutes. The client's blood pressure falls and he may experience syncope. He begins to vomit copiously and may experience difficulty breathing, chest pain, blurred vision, and confusion. The symptoms may persist for at least 30 minutes up to several hours, leaving the client exhausted and weak.

87. 2: When assessing the fetal heart rate with the nonstress test (NST), a normal finding is at least 2 accelerations of at least 15 bpm over 15 seconds for a fetus of ≥ 32 weeks (the normal rate is 10 bpm over 10 seconds at < 32 weeks.) A healthy fetus should exhibit an increased fetal heart rate with movement, and lack of accelerations may indicate hypoxemia or acidosis. However, if a 20-minute period does not show accelerations, the fetus may be in a sleeping cycle, so the testing should be extended to a 40-minute period.

88. 4: The metabolic effect that is most common if a client is taking a loop diuretic is hypokalemia. Therefore, clients are often prescribed supplementary potassium to take with the loop diuretic and have regular monitoring of electrolytes. Other metabolic effects that may occur are hyperglycemia and hyperuricemia. Some people may develop gastrointestinal problems, such as nausea, vomiting, and diarrhea. Other adverse effects include thrombocytopenia, neutropenia, agranulocytosis, headache, tinnitus, dizziness, and blurred vision.

89. 4 milliliters: If an infant is to receive 65 milligrams of acetaminophen elixir that contains 80 milligrams per 5 milliliters, the following formula applies:

$$\frac{\text{desired dose}}{\text{available concentration}} = \text{dose volume}$$

$$\frac{65 \; mg}{\frac{80 \; mg}{5 \; mL}} = 65 \; mg \times \frac{5 \; mL}{80 \; mg} = \frac{65}{16} mL \approx 4 \; mL$$

90. 3: If the nurse is caring for a Hmong client whose death appears imminent and the family members want to dress the client in traditional clothing, the nurse should realize that this is part of a death ritual and assist them in dressing the client as much as possible while treatment is still ongoing. Hmong belief is that people's souls go to the afterlife in the same clothing they wore at death, so the clothing the client is wearing at death may be very important to them.

91. 1, 2, and 5: If a client receiving treatment for breast cancer feels severely anxious, the interventions that are likely to be most effective are to instruct the client in relaxation exercises, such as deep breathing, meditation, or imagery. The nurse should encourage the client to express concerns and take the time to listen to the client as well as attempt to determine what relieves the client's anxiety and what exacerbates it in order to help the client find effective coping mechanisms.

92. 1, 2, and 4: The following ECG tracing represents premature ventricular contraction. If occurring without other abnormality in clients who are otherwise healthy, PVCs are usually of no particular concern and are not generally treated. PVCs may result from intake of caffeine, nicotine, or alcohol. However, frequent PVCs following a myocardial infarction increase the mortality risk and must be carefully monitored. PVCs may also occur in conjunction with underlying supraventricular dysrhythmias.

93. 4: If a dying client's spouse has been teary and obviously grieving for months but seems detached and relatively unemotional when death is imminent, the most likely reason for the spouse's reaction is premature completion of anticipatory grief. The spouse began the grieving process early, anticipating the loss and the emotions, and may be quite spent and emotionally withdrawn when this process completes. A different type of grieving will occur when the client actually dies.

94. 3: If a client is receiving warfarin for venous thrombosis and the client's INR is 4.0 without evidence of bleeding, the nurse should anticipate that the dosage of warfarin will be held or reduced until the INR decreases. The INR level should be maintained at 2.0 to 3.0 for venous thrombosis, pulmonary embolism, and valvular heart disease, and at 2.5 to 3.5 for clients with mechanical heart valves or recurrent systemic emboli. Vitamin K is generally not indicated as a reversal agent with an INR below 5.0, especially with no evidence of bleeding.

95. 3: A common psychosocial response of a pregnant client to pregnancy during the first trimester is ambivalence. Because many pregnancies are unplanned, the client may not feel prepared for motherhood or may feel apprehensive about the physical changes. Multiparas may be concerned about coping with additional children and the expenses involved in raising children. During this first trimester, pregnant women tend to be more concerned about the self than the fetus, especially if they experience morning sickness and/or mood swings associated with hormonal changes.

96. Correct order:

Consciousness
Wakefulness
(1) III. Arousal
Drowsiness
(2) I. Confusion
Inattentiveness
(3) II. Delirium
(4) V. Stupor
(5) IV. Vegetative state
Coma

97.

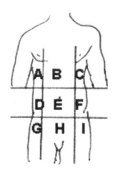

A. Right hypochondriac
B. Epigastric
C. Left hypochondriac
D. Right lumbar
E. Umbilical
F. Left lumbar
G. Right Inguinal
H. Hypogastric/Suprapubic
I. Left Inguinal

98. 1: If a patient with chronic glomerulonephritis has nursing diagnoses of activity intolerance, self-care deficit, excess fluid volume, ineffective self-health management, and anxiety, the first need that should have priority is excess fluid volume because resolving this is a physiological need. Physiological needs always must be dealt with first. The second need to consider is anxiety because being free from anxiety is associated with safety needs, which include the need to have security and to be free of fear and anxiety.

99. 4: If a client engages in yelling and name calling with anger escalating, exhibiting the prodromal syndrome, and the nurse is concerned that the client is at risk of self- or other-directed violence, the initial intervention should be to call for additional help in case the situation turns violent. Then, the nurse can use techniques to try to deal with the aggression, including talking down, giving medication, removing self and others from the immediate area, and using restraints.

100. 3: If a client who has been prescribed oral contraceptives also takes St. John's wort, vitamin D3, calcium carbonate, acetaminophen, and multivitamins, then the nurse should tell the client that St. John's wort should not be taken with oral contraceptives because the herbal preparation increases the rate of absorption of some medications, such as oral contraceptives, decreasing their effectiveness. Acetaminophen, vitamin D, calcium carbonate, and multivitamins pose no problem.

101. 2, 3, 4 and 5: When assessing a neonate's respiratory status, the following are indications of respiratory distress:

- Persistent respiratory rate at rest of > 60 to 70
- Flaring nostrils
- Sternal and/or intercostal retractions
- Grunting expirations

If any of these signs or symptoms is present, then the infant must undergo a thorough assessment to determine the underlying cause. The infant should be assessed for pallor or cyanosis and the lungs auscultated. The child is at risk of aspiration if the respiratory rate is > 60 when feeding.

102. 2: Benzodiazepines are usually avoided in frail older adults because of increased risk of falls associated with common adverse effects of drowsiness, sedation, hypotension, and loss of coordination. Benzodiazepines are frequently prescribed as first-line therapy for relief of anxiety, especially generalized anxiety disorder and panic disorder. Benzodiazepines are also sometimes prescribed for insomnia, although in some cases clients have paradoxical reactions in which the client response is the opposite of that expected.

103. 1: When reviewing dietary restriction with an immunocompromised client following kidney transplantation, the client should be advised to avoid bean sprouts because of the chance they may harbor pathogenic organisms. Clients should also be advised to avoid grapefruit and grapefruit juice, which may interfere with some medications, as well as raw or undercooked meats and uncooked dough that contains raw eggs, such as cookie dough. Clients should also be advised to limit or avoid foods from buffets or salad bars as they may not be properly prepared or may sit for prolonged periods, encouraging the growth of bacteria.

104. 2 tablets: If a client has been taking 112 micrograms of levothyroxine daily, but the physician has changed the dosage to 0.224 milligrams daily, and the patient wants to use up the tablets on hand, the first step is to convert 112 micrograms into milligrams: 1 microgram = 0.001 mg X 112 = 0.112 mg. Then, this dosage is divided into the prescribed dose: 0.224/0.112 = 2 tablets.

105. 2: The first indication of amniotic fluid embolism (also called pregnancy-related anaphylactoid syndrome) is usually sudden onset of acute dyspnea because the amniotic fluid containing fetal debris (meconium, hair, skin cells, vernix) enters the maternal circulation and obstructs the pulmonary vessels, leading to acute respiratory distress followed by circulatory collapse. Because the amniotic fluid is high in thromboplastin, which interferes with clotting, the patient may develop disseminated intravascular coagulation. Maternal mortality rates are about 80% and those who survive often have neurological impairment.

106. 1, 3, 4, and 5: If a physician has prescribed nortriptyline hydrochloride, a tricyclic antidepressant, for a client with postherpetic syndrome who prefers not to take opioids because of a history of substance abuse, the nurse should advise the client to take the medication at bedtime because it may cause the client to become sedated or to develop postural hypotension. Additionally, the client may need to take a stool softener because the drug may cause dry mouth and constipation. The client should be advised to report urinary or sexual dysfunction, common adverse effects.

107. 1: If a patient was in an automobile accident that resulted in what appeared to be a mild head injury and a fractured femur, and telemetry had been normal until the ECG changes occurred, the changes most likely represent sinus bradycardia resulting from increasing intracranial pressure. As the pulse rate falls, blood pressure increases and breathing may become irregular. Sinus bradycardia can also result from hypovolemia, although blood loss should be minimal with a fractured clavicle.

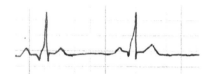

108. 4: Weight at the 5th percentile or lower is an indication of failure to thrive. The next step after physical exam and laboratory work is generally a dietary intake history that lists all fluid and food intake, including amounts and times, for the previous 24 hours and for the next 3 to 5 days, so the child's caloric and nutritional intake can be estimated. While failure to thrive may be an indication of neglect or abuse, many issues must be considered, including health condition, income, health beliefs, lack of parental education, psychosocial issues, and the child's resistance to feeding.

109. 1: Inappropriate affect is a negative symptom. Schizophrenia is characterized by both negative and positive symptoms:

Positive	Negative
Hallucinations (auditory, visual, olfactory, gustatory, tactile)	Affective flattening (poor eye contact, diminished expression, inappropriate affect)
Delusions (persecution, grandeur, reference, control, somatic)	Alogia [poverty of speech] (decreased fluency and content)
Disorganized thinking and speech (echolalia, word salad, incoherence, loose association)	Avolition/Apathy (inability to initiate goal-directed activities, lack of interest in work, grooming, hygiene)
Disorganized behavior (disheveled appearance, restlessness, agitation, inappropriate sexual behavior)	Anhedonia (lack of pleasure in social activities and diminished interest in intimacy)
	Social isolation

110. 3: If a client is to begin hemodialysis, the best option for access is an AV fistula, which is formed by connecting an artery to a vein, usually in the lower arm above the wrist or in the upper arm. The AV fistula requires 2 to 3 months to mature and strengthen before it can be used for hemodialysis, so a client may have a temporary venous catheter placed during this time. An AV graft, which involves connecting an artery and vein with a synthetic vessel matures within 2 to 3 weeks but is more likely to develop clotting or infection than an AV fistula.

111. 3: A client who has been diagnosed with amyotrophic lateral sclerosis (ALS) and uses a wheelchair but still breathes independently may receive palliative care at any time since the client has a life-threatening disease. While hospice care is indicated for client's whose life expectancy is 6 months or less and who are receiving no active treatment, these limitations do not apply to palliative care, which aims to provide comfort measures, such as pain control, and to allow the client to deal with the ongoing stress and needs of severe illness.

112. 1: Indications of graft rejection in intestine recipients are often nonspecific, but beginning signs may be a change in stool output. There are no specific laboratory findings that indicate rejection. Patients may develop fever, abdominal cramping and pain, and vomiting, and the stoma may change in appearance. As rejection progresses, peristalsis may be diminished or absent, and erythema or duskiness of graft may occur. With severe rejection, peristalsis is absent and the mucosa begins to ulcerate and slough.

113. 2: If a client has had a long-leg plaster of Paris cast applied, the cast should be left exposed to the air and not covered because covering it could slow the drying process. The client should be turned with the cast carefully repositioned with the palms of the hands (to avoid making indentations with the fingers) every 2 to 3 hours. A heat cradle with a low-wattage bulb (25 watts) may be placed over the cast or a commercial dryer may be used, but speeding the drying process may result in the cast drying on the outside and staying wet on the inside.

114. 4: Decorticate (flexion) posturing indicates damage to the diencephalon, decerebrate posturing damage to the midbrain and pons, and flaccid posturing damage to the medulla. Comas may be structural or metabolic-induced. Other assessments that may assist in determining cause include assessment of pupillary size and reaction (usually within normal limits with metabolic causes), oculomotor eye movements, and breathing patterns. CT or MRI is also used to identify structural lesions while laboratory testing may identify metabolic abnormalities, such as drug overdose.

115. 2, 4, 5, and 6: If a client who has been taking digoxin presents in the emergency department with an irregular pulse and bradycardia of 22 to 28 bpm as well as complaints of nausea, vomiting, diarrhea, headache, and halo vision, these signs and symptoms are consistent with severe digoxin toxicity. The nurse should anticipate administering digoxin immune Fab to counteract the digoxin. The client should have laboratory tests for digoxin and electrolyte levels (hypokalemia is common) and continuous cardiac monitoring. Supportive treatment should be provided for GI symptoms.

116. 2: If 2 months following allogenic hematopoietic cell transplantation a client has increasing diarrhea, a red rash over parts of the body, and severe generalized itching, and the client's sclerae appear slightly yellow tinged, the nurse should suspect that the client is developing acute graft vs host disease. The typical symptoms (rash, itch, and enteritis) most commonly occur within the first 100 days after transplantation and may progress to chronic graft vs host disease over time.

117. 4: When a client is terminally ill and in the end stages of life, decisions about treatment options, such as providing rehydration, should be based on whether the treatment in question provides comfort and honors the client's wishes. The consequences of treatment or no treatment must be considered. In some cases, if a client does not have an advance directive and cannot express an opinion, the decision about treatment may lie with a healthcare proxy, such as a family member.

118. 2: The best solution for the interstitial cystitis patient who experiences severe burning when emptying the bladder after an instillation is to leave the catheter in place, clamp it for the prescribed period, and then open the catheter to drain the solution. If the patient finds the catheter itself irritating, it can be removed and a second catheter inserted to drain the bladder, but a better solution is to try to change the type or size of the catheter to find one that is less irritating.

119. 2, 3, and 4: If a client with Hodgkin's disease has severe pruritus that prevents him from sleeping and causes him considerable discomfort, the measures that may be most effective in relieving itching include taking the antihistamine diphenhydramine, taking opioid medications, and taking oatmeal baths. However, high humidity and high temperatures tend to aggravate itching, so the humidity is best kept at 30% to 40% and the temperature in the mid to low 60s. Soothing emollients applied to the skin may also provide some relief.

120. 2: A unit of packed red blood cells must be administered to a client within 30 minutes after removal from the blood bank refrigerator. The unit should be examined and returned to the blood bank if gas bubbles or cloudiness are evident as these may be indications of bacterial growth or hemolysis. The cells should be administered slowly ($\leq$ 5 mL/min) for the first 15 minutes, but the flow rate can be increased after that time if the patient has no untoward reaction or is not at risk of circulatory overload.

Thank You

We at Mometrix would like to extend our heartfelt thanks to you, our friend and patron, for allowing us to play a part in your journey. It is a privilege to serve people from all walks of life who are unified in their commitment to building the best future they can for themselves.

The preparation you devote to these important testing milestones may be the most valuable educational opportunity you have for making a real difference in your life. We encourage you to put your heart into it—that feeling of succeeding, overcoming, and yes, conquering will be well worth the hours you've invested.

We want to hear your story, your struggles and your successes, and if you see any opportunities for us to improve our materials so we can help others even more effectively in the future, please share that with us as well. **The team at Mometrix would be absolutely thrilled to hear from you!** So please, send us an email (support@mometrix.com) and let's stay in touch.

If you feel as though you need additional help, please check out the other resources we offer:

Study Guide: http://MometrixStudyGuides.com/NCLEX

Flashcards: http://MometrixFlashcards.com/NCLEX

Made in the USA
Coppell, TX
18 January 2020